Dan-Tien

Dan-Tien–

YOUR SECRET ENERGY CENTER

Christopher J. Markert

SAMUEL WEISER, INC.

York Beach, Maine

First published in 1998 by
Samuel Weiser, Inc.
P.O. Box 612
York Beach, ME 03910-0612

Library of Congress Cataloging-in-Publication Data:

Markert, Christopher, J.
    [Dantien. English]
    Dan-tien—your secret energy center / Christopher Markert
      p. cm.
    First published in Germany as Dantien: die körpermitte als quelle von vitalität und lebensfreude by Irisiana, Munch, Germany, 1997"-
-T.p. verso.
    Includes bibliographical references and index.
    ISBN 1-57863-043-6 (alk. paper)
    1. Hygiene, Taoist. 2. Centering (Psychology) 3. Vital force-
-Therapeutic use. I. Title.
RA776.5.M31513   1998
613--dc21   98-7467
                                              CIP

MG

Cover design by Kathryn Sky-Peck

Typeset in 11/13 Bembo

Printed in the United States of America

04   03   02   01   00   99   98
10 9 8 7 6 5 4 3 2 1

The paper used in this publication meets all the minimum requirements of the American National Standard for Permanence of Paper for Printed Library Materials Z39.48.1984.

Contents

Books by Christopher J. Markert have been published in the USA, England, France, Germany, Holland, Canada, Italy, India, Poland, Israel, Norway, Finland, Spain, Mexico, Argentina, Brazil, and China.

List of Illustrations

Foreword

After reading this book I realized that we can be happy, healthy, and fully functioning only when mind and body harmonize. When the mind is stressed and confused, for example, we experience feelings of displeasure in the body. But when we are happy and fully functioning, we sense pleasure in the body. Luckily this communication works both ways, so that we can attain a happy state of mind by creating a good mind/body balance. This usually happens in a matter of minutes when we use the Dan-Tien concept described here.

The effect is sensational—partly because it is achieved without strenuous exercise, time-consuming meditation or other efforts. The main reason why I find the Dan-Tien approach so appealing is that it can be practiced at any moment and during everyday activities. I did this regularly and enjoyed it (and the pleasure aspect made it even more attractive).

In this way I could easily apply the secret in daily life, and my mind, as well as my body, functioned more joyfully and efficiently. Who would not want to do something that is fun and brings results at the same time?

Gradually I got into the habit of being in touch with my feelings through my body. This made my mind calm, gave me more self-confidence, and generally added to my well-being.

The actual key to this is the ancient Chinese practice of Dan-Tien. It is a method that I highly recommend. At first you may doubt its effectiveness because it is so simple. But any doubts disappear as soon as you give the method the chance it deserves.

—Drs. Wolf van den Hoek

Introduction

The mysteries of the Far East have fascinated me ever since I was a student forty years ago. I felt that here I would discover the secrets that are missing in our Western culture. China has the world's oldest living culture, reaching back over five thousand years. After rejecting its ancient heritage in recent decades, China is now rediscovering its past.

Just as the Chinese are now learning technological skills from us, so we can benefit from the profound wisdom of the Chinese sages.

Over the years I have written two books about this subject that were well-received and widely published.* My version of the I Ching, the "Bible" of the Far East, was even published in Chinese (Mandarin) in Taiwan. The publishers seem to feel that I have a good grasp of the Far-Eastern mentality.

In my present book I describe a more practical aspect of Chinese culture. Western readers will find the concept of Dan-Tien not only enlightening but also very useful in daily life. For me and many others it has been a revelation that changed our lives.

—Christopher J. Markert

---

* *Yin/Yang: the Dynamic Balance* has been published in Germany, France, Holland, Argentina, and Brazil. *I Ching: The Ultimate Success Formula* was published by the Aquarian Press in 1986. It was also published in Germany, Holland, Norway, Finland, Spain, Argentina, Mexico, and Taiwan.

CHAPTER 1

Subtle Signals

Good Feelings are Guiding Us

The secret of good health, happiness, and success lies in the Dan-Tien, according to ancient Chinese texts. Dan-Tien is the source of vitality and joy. We all possess this source, but we are seldom aware of it. We all have an inner compass that leads us to the good life and keeps us in tune with the cosmos. When we listen to its subtle signals we can look forward to a life that is rich and rewarding and blessed with loving relationships.

This compass is so simple and foolproof that we tend to ignore it. Most of us have even been taught to ignore it and to rely instead on complex theories, artificial rules, or belief systems. The concept of Dan-Tien reminds us that all great truths are simple and easily practiced in daily life.

East Asians have known for thousands of years that the core of our vitality and unconscious wisdom lies in our very center. In this area we can spontaneously sense whether we are in tune with life at any given moment. When we think or do something that does not agree with our deepest feelings, we immediately get an unpleasant sensation in our center, in the Dan-Tien. This is a signal that tells us that the way we think or act at this time is not quite right. If we fail to listen to the signal, it will become

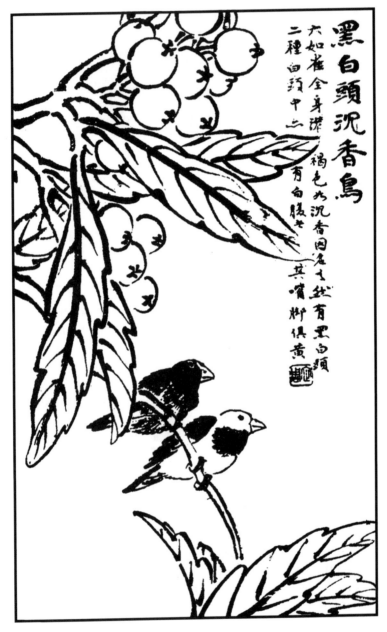

Figure 1. In tune with life at any given moment.

stronger, to the point where we get a "knot" in the stomach. If we habitually ignore the message, we may end up with a stomach ulcer or other psychosomatic complications.

But if we think and act in tune with the Dan-Tien, we notice a pleasant sensation in the belly area. We feel happy and enjoy inner harmony. In time we can learn to cultivate this state, so that it becomes a pleasant habit. Mind and body can thus function optimally and avoid needless stress.

Millions of Happy Minutes

There is a deeper reason why Dan-Tien makes us happy and successful: it connects us with the cosmic life force. When we listen to the signals in our center and act accordingly, we harmonize with the primal force that is called divine. We can find true happiness only when we live in tune with our divine self.

Dan-Tien offers no philosophical systems, moral precepts, psychological analyses, or intellectual explanations. Instead we receive helpful impulses from moment to moment. Just like a child searching for Easter eggs is guided by calls of "warm" or "cold," so we can rely on the hints from our center in our search for happiness and success.

Through Dan-Tien we appreciate and enjoy the "here and now." When we can be happy here and now, when we can enjoy the next minute and the next minute, too, and so on, then we can enjoy the whole day. When we do this all week and through the months, we enjoy millions of happy minutes over the years. It is that simple.

Of course there will be minutes when we notice that something is wrong. Then we feel unhappy until we remember our inner compass and follow its messages. Usually it turns out that we got lost in useless and aimless trains of thought, or perhaps we were doing something that did not fulfill the need of the moment. Instead of living here and now we worried about the past or the future. Instead of sweeping in front of our own door we got involved in other people's problems.

But as soon as we realize that we are on the wrong track, we can change course and restore the good feeling, usually in a matter of seconds or minutes. Our greatest source of happiness is the feeling of being on the right track, here and now. We also feel good when we reach a goal, of course, but we do not reach goals every day.

Divine Impulses

With our inborn Dan-Tien we have a proven system that has been refined over millions of years. It connects us "on-line" with the great cosmic computer. No man-made system can ever match its ingenuity and perfection.

The idea that divine impulses can be relayed through a nerve center in the body does not agree with our Western concepts. We have been taught that the divine can only come from above, through the head, the soul, or the conscience. We have been trained not to trust our "gut feelings" and to suppress our "lower animal instincts." Many people still consider the body below the belt "dirty," unspeakable, or the source of sinful urges.

But in such Western beliefs lies the root of our inability to enjoy day-to-day life. People who reject their body and their emotions are called neurotic. They may get used to their split condition and endure life, but they cannot find real happiness. They can harmonize with themselves and the cosmic whole only occasionally and coincidentally.

They can console themselves with theories or religions that accept suffering as normal, or they can deaden the pain through legal or illegal drugs. They can try to divert themselves with ceaseless activity or noise, but they cannot find access to the secret that their remote ancestors still knew before they were "civilized" through unnatural teachings.

It is possible to drop unnatural habits. We can find our inner center and we can rediscover our ability to enjoy each minute. To do this we need no strenuous exercises or lengthy and costly analyses. All we need to do is trust our inner impulses again and follow them.

In the following chapters we will see how we can practice the secret of Dan-Tien in daily life. But first let us take a look at its ancient origins.

CHAPTER 2

The Ancient Origins of Dan-Tien

The Best Place in the Body

The word Dan-Tien means "belly area," and ancient Chinese texts describe it as "the best place in the body." Sometimes it is also called the One-Point. In Japan it is known as Hara, which simply means "belly."

Taoist teachings reaching back four to five thousand years tell in great detail how to be in touch with the center of vitality and joy, and how to use it as a link with the cosmic power Chi. Taoism is the Chinese folk religion that teaches the "right way," the word Tao meaning "way" or "path." This is not a "father religion" in the Western sense, but a practical philosophy of life with religious roots.

The One-Point is said to be located just below the navel and about an inch inside the body. This point also happens to be just above the womb, the warm and protected place where life originates. Here is the best place for the embryo to grow, where it is safely resting in the gravity center of the mother's body. It is also surrounded by vital organs and has a good, dependable blood supply. Even in the male anatomy, in the absence of a womb, this

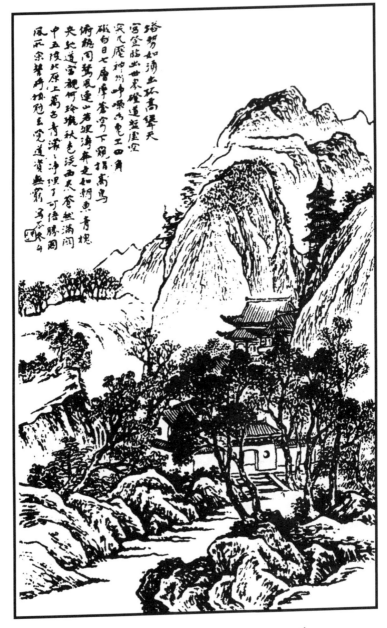

Figure 2. The word Tao means way or path.

is the central core of vitality. While the head, the sense organs, and other external organs are exposed and vulnerable, the One-Point in the belly is a sanctuary, a safe haven, a place where we can feel good.

Persons whose Chi energy is centered in the One-Point are said to be protected from dangers of all kinds. The Dan-Tien can dissolve or "burn" strains, pains, diseases, and other hostile influences. A scattering or loss of Chi energy therefore opens the door to suffering and misfortune, while gathering the life energy in the Dan-Tien brings happiness and good fortune.

Hara, the Japanese One-Point

Zen, the art of emptying the mind and finding the center within, is an experience that cannot easily be described with words. But if Zen has an essence, it might be Hara, the equivalent of Chinese Dan-Tien.

The concept of Hara is deeply rooted in Japanese culture, religion, and daily life. Most Westerners know the word only in connection with Harakiri, the curious way of Japanese suicide. Samurai warriors resort to this way of taking their life because they believe the life energy Ki resides in the belly, not in the heart or the head.

Even today, the Japanese tend to sit, stand, walk, and move in a quite centered way. When they wait in line, for instance, they usually stand firmly on both legs, with a straight spine and relaxed arms and neck. Westerners in this situation would tend to stand "relaxed" on one leg while resting the other, which creates a curve in the spine and a loss of Hara.

The emphasis on a centered posture and attitude is ingrained in the Japanese national character. Persons who are not firmly settled in the Hara tend to be considered immature, unreliable, or confused. Even school children learn about the importance of being centered in the Hara, the "belly brain," in school as well as in daily life.

Most of the Zen meditations have one aim—to clear the mind of irrelevant chatter and to find the true self in the silent center. In the center we experience bliss, while all suffering is only a sign that we have lost touch with our true nature, with Nature in general, and with the cosmic life force Ki.

Westerners who try the path of Zen tend to find the endless "sitting" (Zazen) so boring and painful that they soon give up. In chapter 6 we will return to this subject and show a form of meditation that you will want to do often because it is so enjoyable.

The Dan-Tien Personality

People who live in tune with their center are said to have a "Dan-Tien personality," and this is considered a great honor. They are recognized by their collected, responsible, helpful, and modest attitude. They are self-confident but do not seek the limelight, and they are not interested in impressing or dominating others. Yet they radiate quiet power and attract admirers and followers.

All aspects of their life harmonize with the Dan-Tien, from the smallest detail to their over-all goals. Their life has direction, and they seem to know the meaning of life. They are not afraid of obstacles, enemies, or death. They know that each obstacle can teach them a valuable lesson, and that each enemy is a teacher who can help them to eliminate their weaknesses. They do not fear illness, infections, or bacteria as long as they live in harmony with the universal life force.

They see the good side in every human being and do not exclude anyone. They know that all people like to harmonize with the life force, but many do not know how. When people do not know the secret of Dan-Tien, they easily become angry, greedy, envious, proud, depressed, perverse, jealous, lazy, or sick in mind and body.

Dan-Tien personalities usually look younger and healthier than their age. They can run without losing their breath. They know which foods are good for them and have no problems with digestion or elimination. They know how to gather their energies by sitting in silence with a straight spine. They breathe through the nose, in a quiet rhythm, slowly emptying the lungs with each outbreath. Their eyes are relaxed but alive and mobile, and their voice resonates from the belly. Their nasal passages are clear because the blood circulates freely through the whole body. The head is cool and the feet are warm.

The body movements originate from the center, not from the head or shoulders. There is no fidgeting or nervous finger drumming. Each breath is a joy as well as each step and each movement. Others sense this, and they enjoy the company of the Dan-Tien personality, although they may not be aware of the deeper reasons.

Dan-Tien and Breathing

Taoist masters say that breathing is the driving force for the circulation of the life energy Chi through the body. They know that superficial (upper chest) breathing is the beginning of most diseases. The entire immune system is weakened by poor breathing habits. An amazing number of illnesses and nervous troubles disappear within weeks of adopting the habit of deep breathing.

In the West we know that breathing is necessary to take in oxygen and expel carbon dioxide. But breathing accomplishes many other things that are vital to our health and well-being. With each breath we also stimulate the nerve center in the belly, the Dan-Tien. We notice this when we take a "sigh of relief." Our digestion is also stimulated when we breathe deeply from the diaphragm. Many people suffer from constipation simply because their intestines are not massaged through rhythmic breathing. Even the blood and lymph circulation in this central part of the body depends on the rhythmic contractions of chest and belly.

While the average person inhales 16 to 18 times per minute, the rate goes down to ten or even six breaths after Chi Kung training. It is said that each person is allotted a certain number of breaths at birth. The slower the breath, the longer will be the life. Deep breathing is accomplished by pushing out the air and emptying the lungs after each breath, until the next inhalation follows spontaneously. Slow breathing creates a collected state of inner rest, which in turn reduces the need for oxygen. This state can be further enhanced through meditation practices.

Healthy breathing rises and falls imperceptibly, effortlessly. Above all it is a joy. Whenever we notice that our breathing has become hectic, irregular, nervous, shallow, or unpleasant, we know that something is wrong with the way we think, feel, and act at the moment. In a matter of minutes or even seconds we can feel better by first exhaling and then letting the air rush in. Suddenly the world around us looks a little better. By making this a habit we can change our life.

Our Center of Gravity

Dan-Tien also happens to lie near our gravity center. When we feel good and centered in the belly, this becomes apparent in our body coordination, body awareness, and body movements. All our movements then originate from the center of gravity in our pelvis just below the navel.

In the Far-Eastern martial arts like Judo, Jiujitsu, Kung Fu, and especially Aikido, this idea of centered balance is considered absolutely basic and essential. In past centuries these methods of self-defense were practiced as a matter of survival, not just as games, sports, hobbies, or fitness exercises. The fighter who did not know this secret and thought from his head (instead of the gravity center) moved clumsily and was easily knocked out and killed.

Far-Eastern medical traditions also emphasize the importance of the center, which is at the same time seen as the seat of Chi or Ki, the vital life energy. A person's individual Chi energy is in turn related to the cosmic life force of the universe. To be in touch with this force is said to assure health, happiness, and a long life.

All this may not at first agree with our idea of being an intelligent person with a good head, or a loving person with a big heart. Nevertheless it is a fact that the movements of well-balanced and happy people originate from the hips. This is especially obvious with most children before school age, when they are still moving naturally and spontaneously. We can easily see this when we watch young children at play. If we then watch the movements of "normal" grown-ups, we can see the difference. The average Western adult moves nervously from the head or shoulders, without grace or spontaneous balance.

According to Chinese folk wisdom, a loss of contact with the center is the root of all human suffering and unhappiness. It is also the main cause of psychosomatic illness and the countless "diseases of civilization" that now make up over 90 percent of all our diseases. Unnatural habits of thinking and living destroy the family and spread through society, bringing decadence, hopelessness, hostility, and violence. Only by being in touch with the cosmic Chi through the Dan-Tien can we turn these negative energies into vitality and joy.

Energy Channels

The life energy Chi is said to be at home in the Dan-Tien. From there it circulates in the body through a complex network of channels or conduits, the so-called meridians. The life energy flows freely when we are in good health and feel good. It supplies all organs, tissues, and cells with cosmic life force. Illness begins when the flow stagnates or when there is an excess of Chi somewhere in the body.

Techniques like acupuncture, acupressure, or foot reflexology can be used to stimulate or equalize the flow. Millions of Chinese are also practicing Tai Chi Chuan (shadow boxing) daily to build up and maintain their energy. The proverbial smile of many East Asians is partly explained by their belief that joy and bliss increase vitality, while bad moods, sadness, or melancholy attitudes decrease it.

The art of channeling the Chi energy is known as Chi Kung. Many Chi Kung masters can project their energy to heal sick people without touching them. Others can move inanimate objects at a distance, split blocks of marble with their fists, bend thick iron bars, smash boulders with their bare hands, let cars run over them, etc. These are not legends, but facts documented by Western doctors and scientists.

While practitioners of Western medicine rely almost entirely on technology and the chemicals that they call medicines, healers in the Far East are firmly convinced that health depends on the flow of energy from the Dan-Tien.

We can benefit from this wisdom today. We can keep the energy flowing by loving and appreciating all aspects of our bodily selves. We can resolve tensions by opening blocked energy channels. Whenever we notice that our mind is congested with useless and unpleasant thoughts, we can neutralize them by leading the energy back into the Dan-Tien. Within seconds or minutes we can feel good again and think pleasant, useful thoughts.

The Inner Smile

We can listen to the messages from the Dan-Tien, but we can also cultivate the "inner smile." Taoist masters have taught this secret for thousands of years, and today we can learn it from teachers like Mantak Chia who grew up in Thailand, the "land of smiles."[1]

By practicing the inner smile we create good energy inside us, and we radiate happiness. We dissolve the negative energies such as anger, frustration, and stress. The poisons in our body are neutralized and replaced by honey-like secretions. The immune system is strengthened, and all organs and cells are invigorated.

Instead of paying others to make us happy through artificial entertainment, we create our own joyful reality. We are no longer at the mercy of television, alcohol, or drugs to make us smile. We can smile anywhere and anytime, while we sit, walk, lie, or stand.

Try this now. Lift the corners of your mouth. Then let them drop. Do you feel the difference? Something happens inside you when you smile. You feel good in your Dan-Tien, and gradually the joy seeps into every organ and every cell. As you maintain this sensation you also create good vibrations around you, and people respond to your cheerful attitude.

Just as our inner organs understand the language of the inner smile, so do the people around us. Everybody enjoys dealing with a person who lives in tune with the Dan-Tien.

---

[1] Mantak Chia, *Taoist Ways to Transforming Stress into Vitality* (Huntington, NY: Healing Tao, 1986). He has written many books on Taoism.

The Thai language has a word that comes close to describing this state, *sanuk*. It reflects the charming Thai habit of doing things in a way that makes people feel good. Whether they are at work or at play, they like to do everything with an inner smile. The Thais, being Buddhists, do not believe in an almighty father god, and for their good deeds they do not have to wait for their reward in heaven. The inner smile brings them instant rewards.

The Great Laughter

One Zen student told the story of how he tried to find enlightenment through years of strenuous exercise and self-discipline. He even fasted and tried to do without sleep for long periods.

But instead of finding inner peace he began to feel weak. He suffered from nightmares, he heard strange noises, the blood rose to his head and he had cold feet. He often broke out in sweats, he could not see well and his stomach was upset.

He consulted several doctors, but their medicines did not help. He tried acupuncture without success. Then he heard about a hermit who lived in a cave in a remote mountain area. He was very old and was said to know the secret of health.

The Zen student, who felt quite weak by this time, decided to visit the hermit as a last resort. After walking several days he found the mountain and climbed up to the cave. He respectfully greeted the old man and described his condition.

"I know exactly what is ailing you," said the man, "because I used to be head priest at a large monastery. Many eager young men came to us to find enlightenment. They meditated day and night, and studied the scriptures. But soon they got what I call the Zen disease, because they had allowed their energy to rise to the head. Instead of keeping the Ki in the Hara where it belongs, they had focused it in the mind. This had disturbed their minds and dissipated their energy, and made them feel weak.

"At our gatherings I explained this to them. Then I showed them how to shift the energy back into the Hara and how to exhale through the soles of the feet. When each breath circulates through the whole body down to the feet, body and mind regain their strength.

"When they had practiced this for some weeks, they experienced great vigor and joy. Their complaints and diseases disappeared. They clapped their hands and danced. When they sat in meditation, they often broke out in the great laughter that comes with Satori and enlightenment."

Step by Step

The following chapters show how to get into the Dan-Tien habit easily, step by step. On each page you will find a practical hint or insight that helps you to develop the "right feeling." Gradually you acquire the knack of thinking and doing things that feel good in your Dan-Tien.

These are not intellectual insights, however. Living in tune with the Dan-Tien is a mind-body experience, it involves feelings as well as body awareness. How does a thought feel? How do you experience it in your body? Does it feel good?

As you get into the Dan-Tien habit you gradually drop some ingrained convictions. You discover, for example, that it is quite possible to enjoy everything you think and do. You find that you do not really have to strain and struggle to achieve worthwhile goals, and that your "problems" do not need years of analysis. By experimenting in the coming days you convince yourself that the Dan-Tien approach offers a better solution.

You will not find many formal exercise routines in this book. To be centered and in touch with your Dan-Tien minute by minute is a subtle art that requires improvisation and imagination. This is further explained in chapters 12 and 13, under the headings of "Pleasant and Unpleasant Feelings" (p. 91), "Feel Your Way" (p. 96), and "The Dan-Tien Approach in a Nutshell" (p. 112).

This leaves a final question: Do you really want to be happy? Or has suffering perhaps become a dear habit for you over the years? Do you perhaps feel secure or even comfortable with your favorite pains and problems? Millions of people actually prefer the security of suffering to the scary prospect of being responsible for their own happiness. By blaming others and the world for their misery they can feel superior. They can derive a perverse satisfaction from their unhappiness. In this they are confirmed and justified by certain types of philosophy, religion, and psychotherapy.

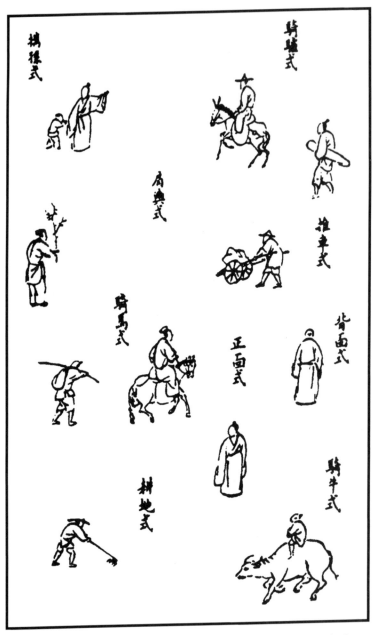

Figure 3. It is the same with everything we think and do each day.

CHAPTER 3

Dan-Tien in Daily Life

The Art of Washing Dishes

The art of feeling good inside can be cultivated. When we wash the dishes, for example, we can do it the hard way or the Dan-Tien way. We can lean forward over the sink with a grim face. We can strain and push ourselves while we hold our breath and count the minutes. We can think about a mistake we made ten years ago. We can envy our neighbor who has the latest dishwashing machine. We can grind our teeth over a remark someone made.

We can also choose to do it the Dan-Tien way. We can balance the body, let each breath come easily, plan our next meal, or enjoy other pleasant thoughts. We can even sing or whistle and swing our hips.

When we wash our dishes the easy way, we feel good inside, our stomach muscles are relaxed. We are in touch with our Dan-Tien, and we are on the right track. If we relapse into tense old habits, we immediately sense an unpleasant impulse in the stomach area. This is a signal to relax and to stop straining. We become aware of a stressed

17

posture, for instance, or of superficial breathing. Now we can get back on the right track and enjoy what we are doing. After the dishes are finished we feel elated, not exhausted.

It is the same with everything we think and do each day.

We can walk down the street and enjoy every step. Or we can push ourselves along with tense shoulders, absent-mindedly dwelling on some unpleasant memory or worry.

We can approach others with determination, a grim face, and tension in our stomach. Or we can relax and be aware of our feelings and theirs. We can sense their needs, while we explain our needs to them. They may not always agree with us, but they will like us spontaneously because they sense that we think and act in tune with life.

Self-Imposed Stress

But most important is the way in which we treat ourselves. We can easily become the victim of self-imposed stress. We can strain and struggle and force ourselves to think and do things we dis-like deep down. We can keep dwelling on trains of thought that make us feel miserable.

Or we can choose the easy and enjoyable life by listening to our Dan-Tien. Our inner compass never fails to point the way. It also knows what we should do first. When we do the thing that is most important at the moment, we feel good inside. But when we waste our time on some irrelevant detail, the good feeling disappears immediately, and we get the message, "Stick to the essentials!" Just as we feel pain when we touch a hot stove, so we feel bad in the Dan-Tien when we think or do things that hinder or hurt our vital interests.

Memories can be another trap if we ignore the signals from our Dan-Tien. Suppose we feel depressed while we think about a past mistake or trauma. The more we picture every detail, the more miserable we feel. We assume, of course, that our depres-sion is caused by the mistake or trauma. Therefore we go on analyzing and digging for solutions, which makes us even more miserable, and so on in a vicious cycle.

But the real cause of all this is not our past. The real cause is our present habit of dwelling on the past in the wrong way. If we had listened to the signals from our Dan-Tien, they would have told us that we were on the wrong track from the beginning. We would have known that it is useless or harmful to dwell on thoughts that can hurt. We would have switched to other thoughts or actions that made us feel good because they served the need of the moment. Or perhaps we would have started to look at our past constructively. All past experiences contain secret lessons or can be used as stepping-stones. Just as there are many ways of washing dishes, so there are many ways of dealing with the past.

The same goes for our thoughts about the future. We can worry about impending disaster and endure the inner strain. Or we can listen to our Dan-Tien and take action that makes us feel good again. We can get busy and prepare ourselves. As soon as we have done this we feel good again, even though there will always be dangers over which we have no control. Worry of any kind tells us invariably that we are ignoring the signals from our Dan-Tien. The message is always, "Don't just worry helplessly, do something right now, or make a decision."

Dan-Tien, the Guiding Organ

Does all this mean that we should throw our intellect overboard and rely on our inner signals only? On the contrary. Dan-Tien helps us to use our mind more effectively, joyfully, and in tune with infinite intelligence.

Figure 4, page 20, provides a way to understand how our mind really works. Each organ does an essential job. The legs enable us to move about, the hands enable us to grasp things, and the external sense organs let us see, hear, smell, taste, and touch.

The brain coordinates nerve impulses, and processes internal and external information. It is an ingenious tool. But it is not the ultimate director and judge. To know what is really and vitally important we have to consult our "gut feelings" that we sense in our vital organs in our very center. This is

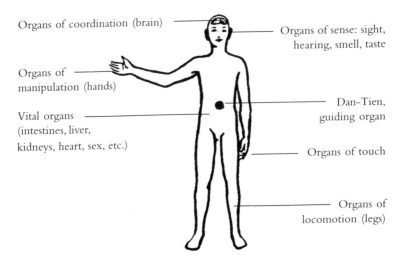

Organs of coordination (brain)

Organs of sense: sight, hearing, smell, taste

Organs of manipulation (hands)

Vital organs (intestines, liver, kidneys, heart, sex, etc.)

Dan-Tien, guiding organ

Organs of touch

Organs of locomotion (legs)

Figure 4. Dan-Tien in relation to the rest of the body.

the point in our mind/body that can tell us at any given moment whether our thoughts and actions really serve our vital needs in harmony with infinite intelligence.

Summary

In our pursuit of happiness and success we need a navigator (brain), and the navigator needs a compass (Dan-Tien). When we feel good inside, our Dan-Tien tells us that we are on course and in tune with life. What we presently think and do makes sense and serves the need of the moment.

Whenever we sense tension or distress building up in our Dan-Tien, our thoughts and actions are off course. Perhaps we are thinking irrelevant thoughts or doing the right thing in the wrong way. Our compass tells us to find a better approach. Now it is time to feel our way until we feel the joy again. This process may sound complicated, but it only takes a minute. Suddenly we feel good again because we harmonize with the Tao, the source of creation.

CHAPTER 4

Diary of a Dan-Tien Student

Getting into the Habit

Until recently very few people in the West knew about Dan-Tien. Even this knowledge did not do much for them if they could not apply the secret in daily life. In my own case it took a year or two until I really got into the habit and reaped all the benefits. Even now I consider myself an advanced student who is gradually perfecting the art.

Some of the changes in my life brought about by Dan-Tien are reflected in my diaries. In this chapter I am quoting from relevant sections that can show the way from theory to practice. At first they may seem somewhat banal. But I think they can illustrate the Dan-Tien way better than most abstract explanations.

October 7

While brushing my teeth I suddenly became aware of tension in my belly. What had happened? I had remembered a nasty televi-

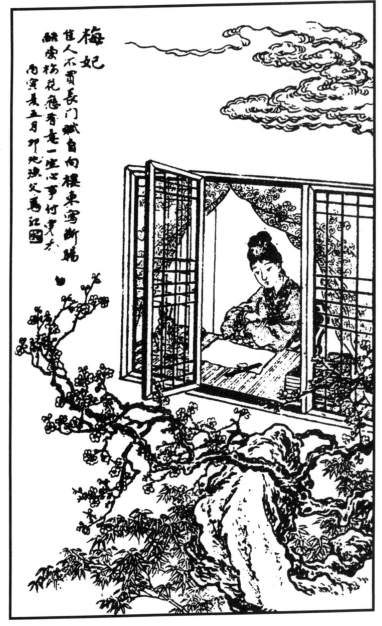

Figure 5. An advanced student gradually perfects the art.

sion program. As soon as I switched my thoughts to another subject that I enjoyed, my body relaxed, and I felt good.

This illustrates that creating happiness can often take only seconds. It is so easy to get bogged down in needless stress for minutes, hours, days, or longer if we are not aware of the signals from the Dan-Tien.

Soon after brushing my teeth I was sitting and reading, when I suddenly felt strained. This time I traced the unpleasant feeling to my left elbow. I had put the arm in a cramped position, and this seemingly irrelevant detail had brought about strain in the mind/body. As soon as I stretched the arm I felt good again. Little things can often make the difference.

October 8

While working on a manuscript I ran out of ideas and felt tense and tired. Should I force myself to go on? I decided that the tension was a signal from the Dan-Tien to relax and use another approach. Therefore I took a nap.

When I woke up I was relaxed, and the writing came easily.

October 9

Today I played tennis. This game has become a kind of Zen exercise for me since I read *The Inner Game of Tennis*.[1] The author, a tennis champion and instructor with Zen and Yoga experience, teaches the art of keeping the mind on the ball. He found that people can improve their game by stopping the mind from interfering with the wisdom of the body. The body knows instinctively where, when, and how to swing the racket. All we have to do is focus the mind on the ball and let the unconscious reflexes do the work. In tennis, as in Zen and in daily life, it is wise to trust our gut feelings (Dan-Tien), to stop the inner chatter, and to think and do what feels good.

---

[1] W. Timothy Gallwey, *The Inner Game of Tennis* (New York: Bantam, 1984).

October 10

On German radio I heard the song "...meide den Kummer und meide den Schmerz, dann ist das Leben ein Scherz..." which means: "avoid regrets, avoid pain, and life will be fun."

I used to find this song silly and superficial, but now I can see the deeper folk wisdom in it. By following the messages of Dan-Tien I also avoid dwelling on sad or painful experiences. Before discovering this secret I used to wallow in painful memories and make myself miserable without finding any answers. I had been encouraged in this by countless psychology books that promised to solve all problems by analyzing a person's past, for years if necessary.

Now I know how to snap out of useless brooding habits almost instantly, simply by trusting my gut feelings and focusing my mind on useful and enjoyable things.

October 12

My goal now is not so much to write a book, but to improve my Dan-Tien skills and keep a record of my progress for future reference. Goals are helpful and necessary, but my first priority is harmony with Dan-Tien. If a goal causes distress in my center, this means to me that I should search for a better goal or a better approach until I feel good again. The end does not justify the means, and a "good" goal becomes "bad" when it is pursued in the wrong way.

In the evening I was invited to join a meeting of spiritually inclined people. There were nine men and women, many of them media and business people. The host of a radio talk show spoke about memory and how to improve it. Then the hostess of the meeting, a journalist, wanted to know what we thought about guidance. Did we all feel that we had guiding spirits or guardian angels or access to the cosmic life force or God? When I explained that I got my guidance from the Dan-Tien, most of the guests found this interesting and agreed that they also followed their gut feelings.

Then the conversation turned to the subject of suffering. Was suffering normal or even necessary for spiritual growth? My theory was, of course, that mental pain shows us that we are on the wrong track, and that we feel good when we think and act in tune with life. In Buddhism, Christianity, and especially Islam, on the other hand, suffering is considered a virtue. The more religious we are, the more we suffer. To me, this sounds like a conspiracy between priests and rulers to keep people obedient, so that they can be more easily ruled and exploited.

I mentioned a parallel between mental and physical suffering. Is it normal and natural to be sick and in pain? Do we benefit from illness because it makes us healthy? I believe the opposite is true—health is normal and natural, and illness tells us that we have deviated from the path of nature. Mental suffering is not only a sickness, it literally makes us sick, it undermines our vitality. How can we lead happier and healthier lives? By listening to Dan-Tien, our inner compass and guide.

Then I pointed out the difference between Hindu and Taoist concepts. Hindus believe in the hierarchy of Chakras along the spine, with the supreme Chakra located on top of the head. This reflects the top-heavy Indo-European mentality, where the mind rules and the body obeys. The Taoist universe is more balanced and centered, with a healthy balance between mind and body, thoughts and feelings, Heaven and Earth. Taoists use their heads, but they are guided by divine impulses through their center, the Dan-Tien. Most of the thousands of Taoist schools of thought agree on this.

October 13

Today was a nice day in Amsterdam, where I am now staying. For almost an hour I enjoyed swinging in the hammock on the balcony that overlooks beautiful gardens. Why do I get so much pleasure from this? Perhaps my remote ancestors were living in trees and swinging from branch to branch. Now my Dan-Tien tells me that this is the kind of setting that makes me feel alive

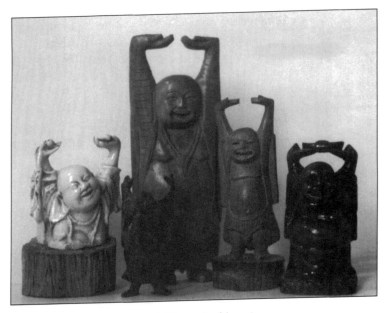

Figure 6. The god of happiness.

and at home. At the same time I can formulate ideas and take notes for a manuscript.

Yesterday I visited a lady, and she asked me if I had a back problem. She had noticed my habit of sitting straight and assumed that I felt uncomfortable. Why didn't I just relax and lean back in the sofa? In recent years I am often asked this question, and I have to explain that I enjoy this posture, that it makes me feel centered and balanced. Sometimes I also enjoy slouching in an easy chair, relaxing in a hammock or reading in bed. But with a straight yet flexible spine, the head balancing on top and the lungs open, I can feel centered in the Dan-Tien.

I have observed that a "relaxed" posture with bent spine and sunken lungs often makes me feel miserable in a matter of minutes. In countries like Japan this is common knowledge, and Yoga teachers keep telling us that the flow of nerve energies gets blocked when the spine is habitually bent. This also affects millions of people today who spend much of the day in "comfortable" chairs watching television or driving cars. Depressed lungs give rise to depressed thoughts of sorrow, fear, anger, blame, etc.

This is why the Chinese god of happiness, who is called *Hotei* in Japan, is pictured in a stretching posture, with a straight spine and open chest.

October 14

While looking through some files I felt a sense of frustration and futility. What was the use of writing all these letters every week, and of getting mountains of mail every year? Why did I waste precious time, energy, and paper in this way?

In previous years such feelings often lingered for days or weeks. Now I know better. I know that they arise when I am thinking or doing the wrong thing at the moment. In this case I felt depressed by a pile of letters because I knew deep down that I had more urgent things to do.

I simply put the file away and focused on the thing that made me feel good in the Dan-Tien because it answered the need of the moment: making an important date for the weekend and getting ready for it.

At other times the opposite might happen. Social engagements might have depressed me because I felt an urgent need to write important letters. In each case the frustration is caused— not by files or dates or whatever—but by the feeling that what I think or do at the time is not urgent.

Later I went shopping, and again I suddenly felt irritated when I looked at the masses of products in the supermarket. Why were there twenty different types of margarine and hundreds of different sweets and chocolates? Why did I eat tons of all this food every year? Why was this mass consumption getting worse every year?

I turned to my Dan-Tien compass for an answer and got this message: First of all, relax your stomach muscles. Second, focus on the thing that you really need most at the moment. Forget about the world's problems and solve your own instead.

As soon as I relaxed my stomach, all other tensions in my body and mind started to drop away. My spine straightened out, my breathing returned to its normal, deep rhythm, and my thoughts returned to useful channels. I composed my menu for the next meal, bought the needed items, and left the supermarket. The problem of mass consumption was still there, but it was not my greatest worry at the moment. Therefore I focused on things of immediate importance, and this made me feel good.

October 15

Last year a more exciting thing happened to me while I was visiting the South Seas. I stayed in a hut on a remote island that belonged to a group called "The Friendly Islands." Although the setting was idyllic, I soon got the "gut feeling" that my luggage was not safe here. I raked the sand in front of my window and, sure enough, there were footprints next morning. After this I hardly dared to leave my hut at all, not even for swimming or buying provisions.

At first I was depressed and felt that my vacation was now ruined. When I consulted my Dan-Tien I got this message: You are unhappy not so much because you might lose your luggage, but because you are worrying instead of acting. Surely there must be something you can do.

But what could I do? I decided to hide my money, passport, and air ticket underneath the linoleum in the hut. For my camera, radio, and walkman I found a secret spot in the grass roof. Then I connected my little electronic alarm to the backpack and went swimming.

When I returned an hour later, I noticed that the alarm had been disconnected by an experienced burglar who had come in through the window. He had gone through all my things, but found nothing of value. My Dan-Tien had saved my vacation, and now it was the burglar's turn to feel frustrated. In the morning I left for another island where the natives were really friendly.

October 16

On this island I took it easy for a while. I also decided to do something about my eyesight, which had suffered somewhat from the stress of the journey. I have never worn glasses due to my habit of doing relaxing eye exercises now and then. Through the years I have derived enormous benefits from the technique developed by an American eye doctor, and I wrote a book about it.[2] The doctor found that most visual defects like far- or near-sightedness are caused or made worse by staring or straining. By relaxing the eyes and the whole nervous system through "swinging," "switching," "palming," "sunning," and other exercises we can improve the eyesight. At the same time we get other benefits that can be even more important. Memory, digestion, general health and well-being improve, for example. We also gain the happy feeling of being in tune with life and the Dan-Tien.

October 17

Years ago I used to wonder why some people had all the luck, while others had to struggle through life. Were some people just born with a sunny disposition? Did they inherit talent or money? Were they more intelligent or better educated? Did they have loving parents or a happy childhood? Did they have a certain philosophy or did they visit the right therapist? Did they play tennis or soccer or belong to the right clubs? Did they practice meditation, Yoga, or aerobics?

Now I know what "lucky" people all have in common. They have a certain knack, an attitude that is easy to spot but hard to describe. They are simply alive in the here and now, they are in touch with life and with their own feelings. They have access to an unconscious source of vitality and inspiration. They think and act more or less spontaneously and are often guided by subtle

[2] Christopher Markert, *Seeing Well Again* (Saffron Walden, England: C. W. Daniel, 1982). This book was also published in the USA, Germany, Holland, and Italy.

hunches. Although they use their head, they also have a kind of gut feeling for what they should do at any given moment. They are usually busy with thoughts and activities that make them feel good.

In other words, they use the secret of Dan-Tien, although they may not be aware of this. They practice the ideas that the Chinese have cultivated since the dawn of time.

CHAPTER 5

Taking Care
of the Dan-Tien

Our Source of Energy and Stamina

People in the Far East get divine guidance through the Dan-Tien. But they are also aware of the down-to-earth aspects of digestion. They take good care of the belly by keeping it warm and selecting the right foods. They know that the digestive tract converts food into energy and gives them the stamina they need in daily life. Their emotional, mental, spiritual, and even social well-being depends on this continuous supply of energy. When their digestion is upset, they know that they will soon feel weak, tired, or irritated, that they will not think and work as well, and that their self-confidence will suffer. Their relationships will be stressed or difficult, and the whole group or family will feel the strain.

On the other hand they know that emotional stress can cause stomach problems, and they try to maintain a balanced state of mind. They also appreciate an even disposition and good manners, and they know the value of quiet moments, silence and meditation.

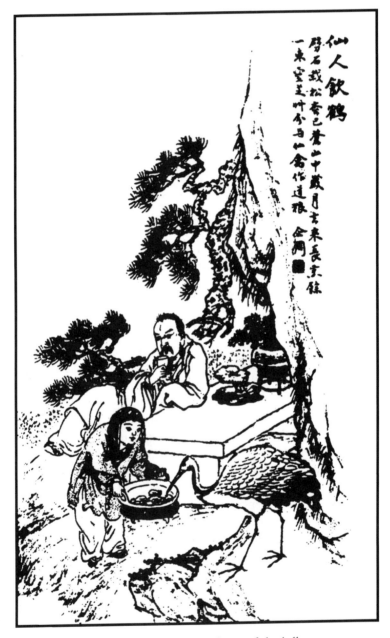

Figure 7. They take good care of the belly.

Whereas Westerners like to wrap shawls around their necks in winter, many East Asians wrap long woolen bands around their bellies, even in the warmer months. In this way they protect the central organs and prevent illness. The proverbial vitality of most Asians can be explained in part by their habit of minding their vital organs.

Quality Food for the Dan-Tien

Westerners tend to pay little attention to the "mind-altering" qualities of food because they believe in "mind over matter." Asians have a better understanding of the interrelationship between mind and body. Farmers' markets in Chinese villages, for example, offer rice, vegetables, and fruit together with medicinal plants. When someone gets sick, a natural medicine is made up in the form of tea, soup, or stew.

Daily meals are looked upon as health-giving compositions that have to have just the right balance, so that they create the right balance in the mind-body. A good Chinese dish is not merely a tasty concoction containing "minimum requirements" of calories, vitamins, and minerals, but a work of art with the right combination of color, flavor, texture, and fragrance. Above all, the ingredients have to be fresh and crisp. Half the art of cooking lies in obtaining first-rate vegetables from the field.

Most people who have been around in the world agree that the Chinese kitchen surpasses all others in variety and finesse. But Chinese restaurants in the West do not often come up to these standards because they rely too much on canned and preserved food.

Chinese meals are not prepared in normal pots and pans, but in "woks," large conical pans suspended over a single flame. Most ingredients are diced or sliced into small pieces, thrown into the hot wok and fried over a strong flame for a few minutes. The meal is then served immediately, while still crisp and fragrant. This method does not only produce tasty and healthy meals, it also saves fuel and time.

But no matter where we are, we can depend on our gut feelings to tell us what is right for us. Deep down we know that we need fresh, wholesome food. At any given moment our Dan-Tien can tell us whether we are really hungry or whether we are just stuffing ourselves because we feel bored or frustrated. We do not need experts to tell us that junk food will undermine our vitality and that obesity is dangerous to our mental and physical well-being. We can learn to distinguish between things that merely taste good and things that make us feel really good inside.

Spontaneous Functioning

When we live in tune with Dan-Tien, we experience our body functions as joyful. We sense that the mind/body harmonizes in all its parts: in the rhythm of breath, in the circulation of blood and the digestive process, in each limb, each muscle and joint, and in each living cell.

But when this feeling of inner union is lost, we tend to see the body as a complex machine, or as a difficult servant who must forever be supervised and controlled. We feel that the body is an inadequate mechanism that must be continuously monitored by experts and specialists, and that it must be improved through miracle drugs, operations, and technology. The mind then plays the role of a dictator who cannot rely on his subordinates and who can never really feel at ease.

This is in fact how modern Western medical science looks upon the body. In the Far East, on the other hand, we find a different belief, which is also shared by atomic physicists. Albert Einstein and Chinese sages agree that mind and body, or spirit and matter, are two aspects of the same thing. Matter is therefore not a passive object that must be moved by an external force. The body is not a passive object that must be controlled by the mind. Natural and divine laws are not externally imposed on the body, but are contained in it.

The body is regulated by its own inner wisdom, which we perceive in the Dan-Tien. The body can also heal itself in most cases if we let it. Hippocrates, the founder of modern medicine, admitted this two thousand years ago: "The doctor can treat a patient and aid the recovery, but only Nature can heal."

Today, the more intelligent doctors all over the world are learning to mobilize the inherent healing powers of the body. They also realize that prevention is better, cheaper, and easier than cure. Unfortunately for the patient, there is no money to be made in prevention. Even well-meaning doctors belong to a system that has vested commercial interests at heart. The powerful medical-pharmaceutical complex focuses on well-paid cures, medicines, and surgery, at the patient's expense.

Chinese Health Insurance

In ancient China it was customary to pay the better doctors a monthly fee for keeping the client in good health. Whenever the client got ill, the doctor had to treat him/her free of charge until health was restored. It was the job of the doctor to detect early symptoms and to be aware of the root causes of disease. In this arrangement, the doctor was rewarded for keeping the client healthy, whereas modern doctors are rewarded when the client gets sick. The sicker the client, the better for the modern doctor and the pharmaceutical industry.

We must realize that our modern health system can be dangerous to our health, and that we cannot expect too much from it. Fortunately we have a better system built into our body, the early warning system called Dan-Tien. When we listen to its signals, we can detect early symptoms and take immediate action.

What is the first faint signal of impending disease? It is the inner unease or stress that we call unhappiness. If we allow this condition to linger until it becomes a habit, it will one day take the form of a physical malfunction. Luckily we can dissolve the inner pain in the beginning stage, before it can cause damage, simply by living in tune with the Dan-Tien again.

Modern medicine is largely disease-oriented. Modern medical books list hundreds of thousands of diseases, with all their symptoms and complications. But they say little or nothing about health and how to maintain it. At the same time it must be admitted that most of the patients have been conditioned to expect doctors to perform quick (and expensive) treatments or repair jobs. Very few people today would be ready to admit that they could have avoided most of their illnesses by adhering to a healthier way of life.

For example, heart attacks and blood vessel degeneration are now the main cause of disease and death in affluent countries. Drug companies are getting rich by developing more and more miracle drugs against this "scourge of modern mankind." The main culprit is said to be cholesterol, and millions of people take expensive drugs to lower their cholesterol level.

People who eat the right foods and feel at peace with themselves because they live in tune with the Dan-Tien seldom suffer from heart disease. Through the habit of listening to the messages from our center we can become almost immune to the number one killer in our society. We can expect to enjoy a long life in good health. Old age can be just as healthy and fulfilling as other stages of life if we remember our early warning system.

According to ancient Chinese medical books, the Dan-Tien can "burn" or dissolve all diseases, at least in the beginning stages. To help in this process, we can now and then retire to a quiet, dark, warm place. There we can spend much time in a lying or meditating position, letting the healing Chi energy gather in the Dan-Tien. Diseased cells in all parts of the body are now located and "burned" by the Chi energy. By actually feeling this and getting into a deep breathing rhythm we speed up the healing process.

The Dan-Tien is said to be so strong that it can handle all poisons without getting harmed. It can dissolve all tensions, mental or physical. When we are facing a threat or an enemy, for example, we can simply relax and "burn" the negative influence. Instead of getting all worked up and starting a fight, we can handle the conflict the easy way.

We will return to the subject of healing in chapter 15.

Keeping the Dan-Tien Happy

Most of us have been told that, to reach a worthwhile goal, we have to strain, struggle, and suffer. Such wisdom may be useful in emergencies, but it does not apply in daily life. In fact, the opposite is true. We accomplish more, learn faster, and think more clearly when mind and body are at ease, when we feel good in the Dan-Tien.

But the habit of straining is ingrained in most of us, and it takes a while to get rid of it. We have to cultivate the art of going with the flow and enjoying each minute. The Dan-Tien shows us the way, it tells us whether we are in tune with life at any given moment. It does not tell us, however, *what* to do. It only indicates if we are on the right track or not. It can only say Yes or No.

Thus we have to use our own ingenuity and imagination to find out what the Dan-Tien is trying to tell us at any given time. This requires a degree of mental flexibility and it takes a while until we get the hang of it. For instance, when I feel uneasy deep down right now, does this mean that I should write a letter, wash the dishes, visit a neighbor, or eat something? The possibilities are endless, and I have to rely on my instinct or intuition to guide me. Rigid rules or logical thinking do not help much here. To stimulate my imagination I can make a list of things that make me feel good. At first I may come up only with the obvious, such as food, pleasant company, or television. But as I become more aware of my real needs, the list grows longer and longer.

It may feel good, for example, to help someone, to sit in the sun, to join a party, to plan the next vacation, to read that exciting book, to walk barefoot in the grass, to smile, to make new acquaintances, to look more attractive, to appreciate a flower, plant, or tree, to buy a gift for someone, to learn a new skill, to sit in the garden, to take a nap, to attend a workshop or lecture, to enjoy a period of silence and solitude, to call someone, to daydream, to visit friends, to go dancing, to sing or do a solo dance, to eat in a cozy restaurant, to remember a pleasant event, to think about the person I love, to go for a walk.

Enjoying the Journey

When we live in tune with our Dan-Tien, we enjoy the path as much as the goal. We can have our cake and eat it, too. Life becomes more pleasant here and now, and it also gains meaning and beauty. We feel as if we are walking through beautiful scenery in nature—and at the end of the path we are once more rewarded with marvelous gifts.

Most religious, philosophical, or psychological systems, on the other hand, involve boring or unpleasant exercises, extensive training, self-discipline, or self-denial. The occasional "highs" tend to wear off and turn into "lows," and the old problems keep reappearing.

Following the Dan-Tien is natural and spontaneous. It is in tune with Nature and therefore with our own nature. There is no need to force ourselves or others or adhere to artificial systems. Once we understand the basic idea, we are on our way, we are on the right track, and we enjoy each step along the way. In fact, there is really nothing we need to learn. We merely have to *un*learn the habit of ignoring our natural impulses and our true nature. By listening to our Dan-Tien, we rediscover our ability to experience the fullness of life, to realize our potential, and to use the opportunities that life offers.

Our Dan-Tien helps us to reach our goals, among other things. But the euphoria of getting what we want seldom lasts. Soon we want something else—such is human nature. Life is a journey, not a destination, and 99 percent of the time we are on our way to some goal. To make our journey worthwhile and enjoyable is just as important as reaching our destinations. By following our Dan-Tien we enjoy every step along the way, and we find satisfaction in our everyday activities, encounters, relationships, and experiences. We enjoy each thought, each step, each breath.

Feelings

What exactly are feelings? Are they located somewhere or are they just wafting through and around us? Are they perhaps in the head, the heart, or all over the body? Or are they just vague and nebulous?

Feelings can give us goose pimples, they can make us blush or sweat. They can be a pain in the neck or a lump in the throat. They can make us feel light or heavy, and they can make our heart beat faster.

But most of the subtle feelings of pleasure or pain arise in the very center of the body, in the Dan-Tien. Whenever we feel really good in this area, we know that mind and body are in harmony. We are then fully functioning, our thoughts and actions flow in tune with life.

When we feel at home in the body, we also feel at home in the world. We enjoy peace of mind and seldom suffer from negative emotions or depressing moods. We see more solutions than problems, more opportunities than difficulties in life. We seem to attract luck and good fortune, we are not accident-prone. We are resistant to disease and have a strong immune system. In the eyes of others we have attractive qualities or sex appeal. We make others feel good because we feel good.

We see good qualities in others and ourselves, we are kind to others and ourselves. We have a loving attitude toward all creation, to Nature, animals, and plants. We are in touch with the cosmic life force or infinite intelligence. We are glad to be alive, we feel good in every limb, every muscle, every cell.

The Secret of Emptiness

Sages and healers in the Far East sometimes talk about the need to attain a state of emptiness. Does this contradict our Western idea of a fulfilling and abundant life? Are we to give up our natural desire to live fully and to use and enjoy each day? What the sages mean by emptiness is the absence of useless or harmful ballast. We can experience the fullness of life only when we are free of mental and physical "garbage."

The story of the Zen master and his student at the tea ceremony illustrates this. While the student chatters away about irrelevant subjects, the master starts filling his cup. He pours the tea until the student exclaims: "Stop, the cup is flowing over!" The master keeps pouring and says: "I am showing you what is going on in your mind. You keep talking and your head is full of confused and useless thoughts. Instead of emptying your mind first, you allow your thinking to become an end in itself. You have forgotten that useful and enlightened thoughts can only arise in the silence of a relaxed and 'empty' mind."

The main cause of mental and physical suffering is our habit of burdening and poisoning ourselves with useless and harmful things. We can be healthy and happy only when we regularly free ourselves from the garbage that tends to accumulate in our mind and body. We can, for example, make sure that we eat only when we are hungry, when the stomach is empty and ready to digest new food; that we exhale all the way before inhaling, so that the used air is expelled and life-giving oxygen can fill the lungs; that we allow the mind to relax regularly and to empty itself of tense ideas and useless chatter, so that our thoughts, words, and actions make sense again. By cleansing mind and body in this way we separate the wheat from the chaff. We get a clear idea of what is really important for us here and now. Our restless intellect relaxes, confused monologues fade away, and we experience life as joyful.

When we get into the habit of breathing deeply and rhythmically, we expel toxic carbon dioxide with each breath, and we inhale the vitally needed oxygen that energizes and rejuvenates. Deep breathing fills us with joy, while superficial breathing depresses us and brings on all kinds of diseases.

When we allow our digestive system to empty and cleanse itself regularly, we feel good. Body and mind can function optimally because no waste products accumulate. Nowadays in the rich Western countries people tend to carry many pounds of sludge in their bowels, which they incorrectly think of as fat. The walls of their intestines are covered with a thick layer of rubbery waste matter, and they can no longer absorb the nutrients from their food. In spite of their overeating they are malnourished and often feel starved. This waste matter also poisons the body and brings on many diseases in the long run, including cancer, arthritis, and heart problems.

The Far-Eastern perspective can show us that abundance and wealth can make us happy only if we understand the secret of "emptiness." The two concepts of "empty" and "full" relate to each other like Yin and Yang, the two elements of the cosmic life energy: they need and complement each other. If we glorify one pole and reject the other, we are bound to become sick and unhappy. We can lead a full life only if we appreciate both sides of the coin, as in the polarity between thoughts and feelings, tension and relaxation, theory and practice, male and female, heaven and earth.

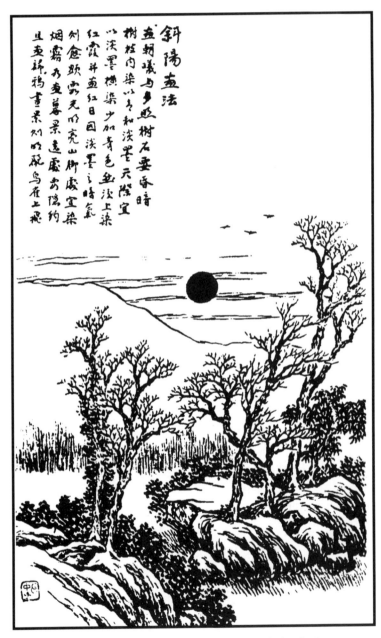

斜陽畫法

畫朝暾與夕照樹石要昏暗
樹枝內染以赭和淡墨天際宜
以淡墨橫染少加青色為淡上染
紅霞並畫紅日圓淡墨之時氣
刻愈歟容光明充山腳霧宜染
烟霧夜麥暮景遠慮宜隱約
且求歸禽畫景刻如歸鳥尤上飛

Figure 8. We can cultivate the Dan-Tien habit further.

CHAPTER 6

Fine-Tuning
the Dan-Tien

Our Quiet Center

We can cultivate the Dan-Tien habit further through a daily routine known as meditation. All Far-Eastern sages agree that "sitting still" for a short period every day brings enormous benefits. Meditation allows us to center and balance the mind/body under optimal conditions.

We can also be centered during everyday activities at home and at work, while washing the dishes, operating a machine, or talking to others. But while we are busy in this way we tend to focus on the periphery and not the center. We are easily dominated by stimuli from our five senses or by our thoughts. There is nothing wrong with thinking, of course, or with seeing, hearing, touching, smelling, and tasting. But these functions should not dominate our life. They should be servants, not masters. All these peripheral activities should be guided by the center, the Dan-Tien.

When this is not the case, we immediately sense that there is something wrong, and we feel unhappy. We can feel good only when our thoughts and our five senses function in harmony with the Dan-Tien. Our thoughts can only be useful, meaningful, and creative when they are fed by the source; they can only flower when they are nourished by life energy from the root.

There are countless meditation techniques to choose from, some of them better than others. Most of them are done in an upright sitting position

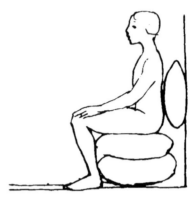

Figure 9.
Comfortable sitting posture.

with crossed legs. This Buddha posture is not easy for most Westerners, and it is not absolutely necessary. Any sitting posture will do, as long as it is not slumping. The spine should be straight, the lungs open, and the head should balance on top. A comfortable chair is all right in the beginning, until the habit is established. Later it is better to use three firm pillows arranged on a bed or soft surface. Two pillows form the seat, and the third one serves as a backrest against the wall. Advanced students use a low stool without a backrest.

Lazy Meditation

Buddha, the great meditation teacher, is sometimes pictured in a lying position. Taoist masters recommend lying down and breathing through the body as an ideal way of relaxing and finding the center. They even claim that this simple and enjoyable routine ensures good health, abundance, and a long life, if done consistently over the years.

You can try it out today. This evening, while lying in bed, take a few minutes to get back into your body. All day long you have been preoccupied with your surroundings and your thoughts. Now you are going to shift your attention down into your body, into your gravity center around the belly and into your legs and feet. You allow your mind/body to get back to normal, after a restless day. At the same time you get into an even, deep breathing rhythm. All this you can do easily, pleasantly, and simultaneously by "exhaling through the soles of your feet."

First you lie down comfortably on your back, with arms by your sides and legs stretched out. Your eyes are closed and you enjoy the feeling of peace in body and mind for a minute. If you feel sleepy, just doze off. Try again some evening when you are less tired.

If you feel like going on, become aware of your breathing. Then, with your next outbreath, visualize your breath slowly flowing down through your whole body, down your legs, and out through the soles of your feet. Picture how the breath streams through all the organs along the way, through the neck, heart, lungs, liver, intestines, kidneys, sex organs, upper legs, knees, calves, and feet.

When your lungs have expelled all the air, the inhaling follows by itself. When your lungs are full again, exhale in the same way through the whole body, down to the soles of your feet, and so on. Do this for several minutes, until you feel thoroughly relaxed, centered, and happy and then doze off. You can do this any day, even for years, as long as you enjoy it.

Mental Pictures

Close your eyes for a moment and picture a juicy ripe peach. Touch the soft, silky skin, let your eyes wander over the round shape, then bite into it, have another bite, and another. Now start chewing and swallowing the delicious juice. Did you notice how saliva collects in your mouth, how your tongue begins to move in anticipation? Can you imagine how your stomach begins to secrete the juices needed for digestion?

Open your eyes again. You have just had a mouth-watering experience by eating an imaginary peach. Your mind was involved and so was your body. By using a strong mental picture you have influenced your body and your mind, and you have even activated your digestion.

You can also use the power of mental pictures in your meditations. Best suited for this are simple black shapes that you have often seen before, such as letters and numbers. Flowers would be more cheerful to look at, but they are not as easily visualized, due to the complex shapes and shades of colors. With closed eyes you can easily picture the letter "A," but to picture a red rose takes effort. In the following meditation you want to use easy images to become centered in a relaxed way.

The Zero Experience

Now you are ready for the visual experience. You are sitting in a comfortable upright position. The light is subdued and you have made sure that you will not be disturbed. Your posture is relaxed, and the head rests easily on top of the spine. The breath comes easily; you emphasize each outbreath, and then let fresh air flow in by itself. You enjoy the silence. Thoughts come and go. Your eyes are closed.

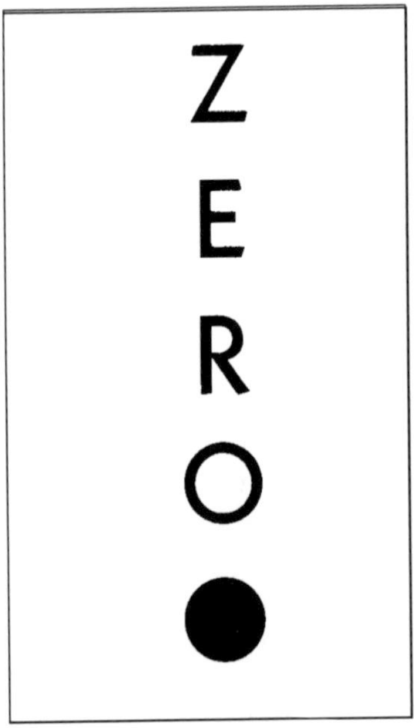

At this point you begin visualizing the letters of the word ZERO, one after the other. First you see the letter "Z." With the next outbreath you let your eyes wander over this shape, following the lines slowly. Do this until your lungs are empty, then let the air flow in by itself.

With the next outbreath you picture the letter "E" below the "Z," and you repeat the cycle. Slowly let your eyes trace the lines of this letter until your lungs are empty. Then let the air rush in by itself and start visualizing the letter "R" below the "Z" and the "E."

Figure 10. The Zero Technique.

Now you take an imaginary thick felt pen or marker pen. Underneath the "R" you draw a thick black "O" with your pen as you exhale slowly. This letter "O" can also be seen as a zero. Once again your eyes slowly trace this shape.

When your lungs are empty, you take your imaginary felt tip pen again. With the next outbreath you begin to fill the round empty space of the "O" with black ink from your pen.

Keep your eyes mobile and relaxed—do not let them stare. Let them wander over and around the black dot that you have just created. The blacker you see the dot, the more relaxed you are, and the better you will feel. When you see the dot in deepest black, you will experience bliss and joy flowing though you, especially in the Dan-Tien.

This is one easy way of centering the mind/body. When you do the Zero Experience the first time, you may not get optimal results, but in any case you should find it enjoyable. If you do not enjoy it, do the "Exhaling Through the Soles of Your Feet" for a few weeks, until you have dissolved the stress.

After you have done the Zero Technique a dozen times, you can also use other words if you wish, such as ENJOY, RELAX, QUIET, CLEAR, UNION. Choose pleasant words and add the "O" at the end, so that you get the black dot effect. In ancient Sanskrit texts, the black dot symbolizes union and origin, the point in which everything is integrated and centered (bindu). In Taoism the black dot is used as a symbol of Tao, the "Way of Nature," or the cosmos.

The black dot also serves as an indicator of your state of mind. You will discover that you cannot picture the dot really black when you are nervous or confused. When you come home from a stressful day, for example, you may only be able to see a circle or a gray dot. But whenever you feel good and centered in the Dan-Tien, you see the dot right away, in deepest black and sharp contours. At the same time you experience the deep joy that comes with inner union.

A Thousand Benefits

Whenever we are in touch with our center we have access to the source of all true riches. Everything we really need tends to come to us in mysterious ways. The feeling of inner fulfillment seldom leaves us. Now and then we may still experience short periods of confusion, but this does not really upset us, because we know that we have access to the universal force. We feel safe in the knowledge that we can always find our way back into this harmony, by listening to the Dan-Tien or by using the techniques described above.

The minutes we spend centering ourselves are the most productive minutes of the day. While we are sitting or lying there, seemingly idle and unproductive, our thoughts, plans, and projects crystallize around our central purpose. Suddenly we know what to do first and how to go about it. The coming day organizes itself into a more efficient pattern, so that we accomplish more with less effort.

Even the body functions more efficiently and becomes less disease-prone. The self-healing forces take effect and begin to correct strains, imbalances, and abnormalities. The senses of sight, smell, hearing, taste, and touch become more acute. All bodily functions, including digestion, elimination, blood circulation, blood pressure, heartbeat, and breathing, begin to normalize.

In our daily activities we become less often fatigued. Mind and body function together toward a worthwhile goal. During hectic periods we accomplish more with less strain because the mind is focused. Fatigue only sets in when we lose our focus, when our thoughts, actions, and body movements become aimless. What wears us out on a normal day is usually not the work itself, but the inner strain and confusion. But as soon as we think and act from the center, we relax, we know exactly what to do, and everything falls into place.

The Short Route to the Goal

There are many ways and paths to the state of inner union. There are also many methods that have been developed into elaborate systems that require years of thorough training. Even after years of such effort, the student can never be sure of reaching the goal.

Many teachers, gurus, and therapists actually have a vested interest in drawing out the learning process, to increase their own importance and the students' dependence on them. They may not be consciously aware of this ulterior motive, but they enjoy the social position and/or the material and other rewards.

The Taoist methods described in this book offer a shorter and easier route to happiness and success. They contain the accumulated folk wisdom of thousands of years. They are simple but practical. To find Dan-Tien we do not have to understand complex systems or abandon life in the real world. We do not have to meditate for hours or quit working. We do not have to search for a spiritual master in the Himalayan mountains. Although such a journey to the East can be an enlightening experience, it is not really essential. The guide we are looking for is in ourselves, in the Dan-Tien.

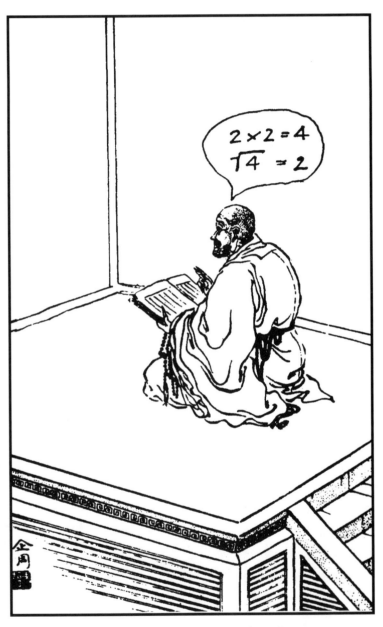

Figure 11. We in the West can also cultivate
this subtle awareness and benefit from it.

CHAPTER 7

Dan-Tien:
A Western Explanation

Far-Eastern Wisdom and Western Logic

Dan-Tien is a Chinese concept that has no equivalent in the West. Yet the principle of Dan-Tien is universal, it applies to human beings everywhere. People in the Far East may be more aware of subtle feelings, but Westerners can also cultivate this awareness and benefit from it.

In the West we have been more interested in science and in dominating the environment. The law of gravity was discovered by Isaac Newton when he watched an apple fall from a tree. Although this was an English apple, the law of gravity also applies in China and elsewhere.

Since the days of Newton, the Chinese have learned to cultivate Western ways of using science and technology. At first they were suspicious of the Western devils with their strange machines, but now they use this technology with great success.

In the same way we in the West can learn from Far-Eastern wisdom. But it would be a mistake to accept strange beliefs blindly and to superimpose an alien concept on our Western culture. To get the full benefits we have to integrate and digest the new ideas. We have to adjust or correct our old beliefs where they are found to be narrow or unrealistic. We must eliminate weaknesses and blind spots in our picture of the world.

One such weakness is our habit of ignoring subtle feelings and of worshiping the intellect. We are very good at using logical reasoning to the point where it hurts and defeats its purpose.

Yet there is no real conflict between intellect and intuition, between Far-Eastern wisdom and Western logic. We can use our Western intellect to explain Far-Eastern concepts like Dan-Tien. We can arrive at a true synthesis that will be very useful not only for us but also for people in the Orient. Their wisdom is often obscured by irrational superstitions that need to be cleared up by logical thinking.

The Anatomy of Dan-Tien

A Western medical doctor might explain the Dan-Tien phenomenon by relating it to the nervous system. The human body has two main nervous systems. One coordinates the body with the environment. The other has the job of maintaining essential life processes inside the body. In lay terms we could simply speak of an inner and an outer mind.

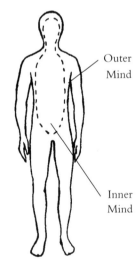

We think with the outer mind, and we are proud of our intelligence. But our liver, for example, is incredibly intelligent. It can maintain over one hundred chemical processes simultaneously, and produce several vitamins besides. Of Napoleon it is said that he was so brilliant that he could

Figure 12.
Outer and inner mind.

do three things at the same time. Today we know that his liver was even smarter than his brain.

Outer Mind: Largely conscious, it deals with the environment and solves external problems. It reacts to unpredictable external events through fast, simplified decisions and aggressive or defensive action. It is by nature alert, assertive, logical and decisive. It perceives events in logical sequence, using memory and imagination. It acts through the five senses (sight, hearing, touch, taste, and smell), limbs (hands and feet) and extensions (tools, mental tools, language, knowledge, culture, etc.).

Inner Mind: Largely unconscious, it maintains life through metabolism, digestion, growth, healing, and reproduction. These gradual biological processes are so complex that they can take place only in a controlled and favorable internal environment and in a largely automatic manner. The inner mind is therefore by nature patient, slow, and peaceful. It perceives events not in logical sequence, but in all-encompassing pictures. Much of its work is done during sleep, and dreams are an example of how it experiences reality.

It acts through the central vital and digestive organs and glands. Some of these activities can be consciously perceived by the outer mind, for example through "gut feelings" in the belly area.

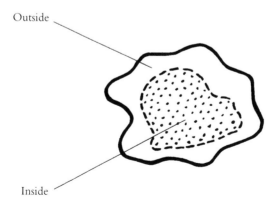

Figure 13. The Amoeba.

The Origin of Life

This inside-outside arrangement (figure 13, page 53) is found in all living things, by the way. In its simplest form it can be observed in our remote ancestor, the amoeba. All organic cells consist mainly of an inner core and a protective surface layer.

Outside: Protects the inner core. Sensitive to light, chemicals, electric currents, pressures, etc. Lets in nourishing substances and keeps out harmful matter. Makes simple decisions.

Inside: Maintains life process, converts energy and takes care of reproduction through cell division.

Biologists agree that, millions of years ago, the first organic cell contained the basic model for all later creatures: plants, animals, and humans. Larger organisms are huge conglomerates of cells that have united for survival. The various cells then specialize in certain functions such as movement, communication, feeding, and reproduction.

Our Glamorous "Outer Mind"

All our thinking takes place on the superficial conscious level of the outer mind. Naturally we tend to think that our conscious mind is more important than the unconscious inner mind. We think that the human brain is the crown of creation, and that we can solve all problems through logical reasoning. We tend to ignore our feelings and despise the body functions. The result is unhappiness, suffering, and sickness of mind and body.

But there is no need to stop thinking or to throw our intellect overboard. Our brain can be very useful—but only if it harmonizes with our feelings. And the simplest way to attain this harmony is through the Dan-Tien, which gives us a direct line to our inner mind. There are many other ways of reading our feelings, but all of them are somewhat difficult, complicated, or impractical. Some of them create more problems than they solve.

When two equally complex systems depend on each other for life and well-being, the question of importance becomes irrelevant. Each is important in its own sphere. The outer mind acts as the leader in most external matters, while the inner mind is in charge when it comes to internal matters. The outer mind may be more visible and "glamorous" because it stands in the limelight of consciousness and often makes spectacular external decisions. But it certainly could not exist without the support of the inner mind.

Psychologists, philosophers, and priests have argued about the "mind/body problem" for thousands of years. They have asked: "Did the mind or the body originate first? Which of the two is better and should rule the other? Can the mind exist without the body?"

All such questions answer themselves when they are related to the biological model described here. But almost all Western philosophies and religions, including Freud's theories, stress the superiority of the outer mind. They state that the body and the emotions cannot be trusted because they are primitive and chaotic, or that they are the source of all evil. Some of them (including Descartes) even believed that we would be better off without the body.

The Alienated Intellect

When people lose touch with their center they often feel hostile toward the body, and alienated from nature and life in general. They have lost access to the comfortable central world where things function by themselves, where nature supports them, and where healing and regenerating powers take effect. They cannot really feel at home anywhere, and anything they think or do is somewhat out of tune with the cosmic order.

Especially in the modern cities today, they are exposed to a hectic, man-made, fast-changing scene, to the incessant barrage of the mass media and to general over-activity. In many households one or more television sets are turned on most of the day and night.

In such artificial surroundings, people can easily lose touch with the other world, the comfortable, natural world of the "inner mind." Loneliness and emptiness is what they experience when they are alienated from the inner self. Life becomes meaningless and unbearable.

In their desperate attempt to kill the pain and to feel happy again, many of them reach for the bottle. Others resort to legal or illegal drugs. They grew up in a drug-oriented society where it is considered normal and natural to depend on chemicals to stimulate, tranquilize, kill pain, induce sleep, or create a happy state of mind. But by using such crutches habitually they only multiply their problems.

When the intellect ignores or suppresses the Dan-Tien, it acts like a dictator. Like all dictators it can then claim some initial successes. But in the long run it must fail because it lacks the support of its power base.

Successful leaders stay in touch with the people; they have a gut feeling for what the people need and want. They enjoy a happy, dynamic interrelationship between the top and the bottom of society.

The Lowly Body

We generally picture the mind as being "higher" than the body. We tend to look up to the mind and down on the body. The high is superior and the low is inferior. This at least, is how our conscious outer mind sees it. But if our unconscious inner mind could talk, it would say the opposite. It would complain about the impatient and arrogant conscious mind "up there."

"There is nothing either good or bad, but thinking makes it so," said Shakespeare.[1] Whether we like something or not depends on our point of view. Our inner mind, for example, prefers the low and protected places where it can best fulfill its biological functions comfortably and undisturbed. Our outer mind, on the other hand, prefers the high and exposed places from which it can overlook and control the environment.

Once we become aware of the bias in our thinking, we can appreciate the body for what it is. We realize that the Dan-Tien

---

[1] William Shakespeare, *Hamlet,* 1. 259.

is below the belt for good reasons. We also realize that the mind is "good" only when it harmonizes with the body, and that it is "bad" when it does not.

People who idolize the high at the expense of the low will also tend to be nervous and arrogant much of the time. They will feel uncomfortable with sex, women, and children. They will look down upon life on Earth as opposed to life in Heaven. Most likely they will prefer male values to female values, and picture the cosmic life force as a male entity. The ancient Chinese had a more balanced concept. They believed that the life force Chi is composed of the male and female elements, Yang and Yin. This is why they were in touch with their feelings and aware of the Dan-Tien, as we shall see in the next chapter.

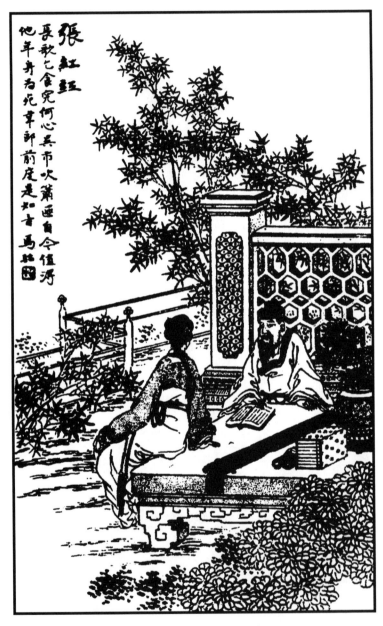

Figure 14. The Yin/Yang polarity
determines the relation between the sexes.

CHAPTER 8

Yin and Yang, Female and Male

The Yin/Yang Balance

For thousands of years the Chinese have believed that they can be happy, healthy, and successful only when they harmonized with the life force, Chi, through the Dan-Tien. Chi, in turn, is composed of Yin and Yang, the female and male elements. The Yin/Yang polarity rules not only the relation between the sexes, but also the balance between other polarized units, such as mind and body, conscious and unconscious mind, spirit and matter, Heaven and Earth, right and left, above and below, ideal and reality.

Both poles have equal value, they need and complement each other. But both become destructive and malevolent when the subtle balance between them is disturbed. Our aim is therefore not to favor one or the other pole because it seems "better," but to favor a balance that will enhance both poles.

This is where Far-Eastern thinking often differs from our Western concepts. The Chinese with their ancient culture seem to have developed a sense of balance and a sense of humor that most of us lack. The very fact that we have no Western equivalent for the Yin/Yang concept demonstrates the blind spot in our culture. We are still amateurs in the art of finding a sane balance between man and woman, thoughts and feelings, mind and body, logic and intuition, father and mother, Heaven and Earth, spirit and matter, tension and relaxation, etc.

Very few Western thinkers seem to have noticed this gap until recently, but a growing number have become aware of it within the last decades. Ralph Waldo Emerson was one of the first to deal with the subject. In his "Essays" he spoke of the polarity that we can see everywhere in nature, in spirit and matter, man and woman, subjective and objective, inside and outside, above and below, yes and no, etc.

Emerson shared the Far-Eastern belief that the two poles complement each other and that they are both equally important. Most Western philosophies and scriptures, on the other hand, glorify one pole and neglect or reject the other. For instance, they think of the mind as better than the body, thoughts better than feelings, Heaven better than Earth, the "Heavenly Father" better than the "Mother Earth." Our culture worships male values and degrades many of the female values.

Here lies the main reason why so many Western women reject the female role: they sense that their female qualities are considered inferior in our Yang-oriented culture. But because they are themselves part of this society, they try to acquire male qualities, they try to be "as good as men or better." Instead of being proud of their femininity, they suppress it even further. Although the Chinese culture is not free of sexism, it is more Yin-oriented as a whole.

The Yin/Yang concept can help us gain a healthier balance between the sexes and a more sane attitude toward the body and our feelings. Our subtle feelings are by their very nature more "feminine" than "masculine." Men as well as women must cultivate their Yin qualities as much as their Yang qualities if they want to be real human beings. The simplest way to do this is to live in tune with the Dan-Tien. Everything falls into place when we get into the habit of listening to the messages from our center.

Harmony Between Men and Women

A kingdom in ancient China was in turmoil, and the king was desperate. His people lost confidence in him, the officials were corrupt, and crime was everywhere. Finally he consulted a wise old man who lived in the mountains, and he received this advice:

"To straighten out your empire you must first create order in the provinces. To have good government in the provinces you must see that there is harmony in the towns and villages. The people in the towns and villages can only be good if their families live in harmony. Order in the family is only possible if there is harmony between man and woman. Men and women can only love and understand each other if they know about Yin and Yang.

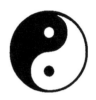

Figure 15.
Yin/Yang Symbol

"The Yin/Yang symbol (figure 15) shows the two elements that embrace each other in a continuous flowing movement. It shows duality and polarity in a unifying circle. Each pole furthermore contains the seed of the other and shares certain qualities with the other. This is why they can understand and complement each other. The whole empire rests on the love and understanding between man and woman. This harmony cannot be created by edicts, laws, police forces, or armies. It can only be inspired by a king who lives in tune with the cosmos through his Dan-Tien and knows the secret of Yin and Yang."

The basic meaning of the Yin/Yang polarity is usually described as shady/sunny, gentle/firm, sweet/salty, etc. Yang is often pictured as a winged dragon that roams the heavens and initiates things. Yin is often represented as a mare, graceful, fertile, capable of giving and maintaining life. When Yin shows its undesirable aspects, it becomes shapeless, passive, chaotic, shady, negative, nagging, hysterical, and small-minded. It can lose the wider perspective and waste its time on petty details and routines.

When Yang shows its undesirable aspects, it becomes rigid, arrogant, aggressive, fanatical, impatient, top-heavy, cruel, sterile, and lonely. It can lose touch with reality and the Earth; it can waste energy on fanatical schemes and lofty ideals.

These undesirable qualities usually emerge in Yin and Yang simultaneously when the balance between them is disturbed. For instance, Yin will tend to become chaotic and negative as soon as Yang becomes rigid and arrogant. Or Yang will become impatient when Yin is too passive.

When people are confused about their own Yin/Yang balance, they must also be confused in their relationships with the opposite sex and their own sex. They feel insecure in the spectrum that lies between friendship and sexuality. This happens invariably when people lose touch with their center. But the confusion disappears as if by magic when they listen to the messages of their Dan-Tien again.

Yin and Yang each have their strong and weak points, and this is why they need and complement each other. In some translations of Chinese texts, Yang is described as "creative" and Yin as "receptive," implying that the male is the source of life that uses the female as a passive tool. This idea corresponds, of course, to our Western image of the male god who creates the universe without female help. Yet the Chinese language has no word for "God." It only speaks of Chi, the Absolute, which manifests itself as Yin and Yang. The Chinese word that comes closest to our concept of God is Yang, the male half of creation.

Westerners are in effect worshiping half of creation and ignoring or suppressing the other half. This single-minded approach has brought us much success in the areas of science, technology, and warfare. But it is also responsible for most of our frustrations and neuroses, for our artificial way of life, and our declining vitality. The typical Westerner is so preoccupied with the external success that he/she has no time left to listen to the subtle cosmic messages in the Dan-Tien.

The Differences Between Men and Women

Women are Yin creatures with a touch of Yang. Men are Yang creatures with a touch of Yin. Nobody is 100 percent male or female, and nobody feels comfortable in narrow sex roles. We can only feel good as men or women when we are true to our true nature.

Yet every child knows that men are different from women. The main difference is plainly biological. A woman can bear children. She carries a child for many months during pregnancy and lactates, feeds, and cares for it several years afterward. During this time she is quite vulnerable and dependent on the security and food supply that is normally provided by a male. When a woman brings up her child without the benefit of a husband, she needs the help of relatives, friends, or institutions.

People who insist that there is really no difference are perhaps right with regard to their own personalities, but they do not speak for the majority. Most people see the following differences:

❦ Girls mature sooner, feel attracted to boys earlier.

❦ Boys reach puberty later and get interested in sex later.

❦ Women tend to be more efficient and "energy saving" in their behavior, and more graceful in their movements. In their appearance they like to emphasize vitality and vivacity (healthy skin, shiny hair, shapely figure, lively personality).

❦ Men tend to exert more energy in their activities and body movements. Their appearance and clothing tend to be more functional and utilitarian.

❦ Women tend to think from the bottom up; they feel first and then think about it.

❦ Men tend to think from the top down, they think first and then get emotionally involved.

❦ Women like to communicate continuously. They talk as they think, spontaneously and effortlessly, sometimes about trivial matters.

❦ Men like periods of silence, after which they come out and say something "logical" or radical. They need time for thinking.

❁ Women tend to devote themselves to a person whom they like or love, even in business or politics, and to accept that person's ideas. They are more subjective.

❁ Men tend to work for a cause, idea, or organization, rather than a person. They are more objective.

❁ Women tend to progress steadily, efficiently, relaxedly, and have less need for periods of total rest.

❁ Men tend toward gigantic efforts, they go after big goals, waste much energy, and then have to rest.

❁ Women are more involved in a network of relationships; they usually write more vacation post cards and Christmas cards.

❁ Men tend to take relationships for granted and forget the little attentions, anniversaries, and gifts.

❁ Women tend to express themselves more cautiously, in more ambiguous and pleasing ways. They look people in the face and try to read their thoughts.

❁ Men tend to use stronger and more assertive words, even if this offends people. Their eyes turn to some distant point while they explain "the truth."

❁ Women read faster and remember more of what they read. Their intellect screens out less of the input, it is more open and less decisive.

❁ Men read more slowly, they screen and cross-examine every statement, and remember only what they find important.

❁ Women's brains are smaller and finer, and the two brain hemispheres are more closely connected. This enables them to think "with feeling" and to see the connection between seemingly separate ideas.

❁ Men's brains are larger and more coarse, and their feelings are more separated from their thoughts. This enables them to pursue their goals more single-mindedly or fanatically.

Men and women neglect these basic differences at their peril. If they compete with the opposite sex and try to invade each other's territory, they may waste much time and accomplish little. To trade roles now and then can be fun, but to lose one's own sex identity entirely and to aspire to the unisex ideal is no solution for most people.

Sex confusion arises only when people lose touch with their center. But when the Chi energy is centered in the Dan-Tien, people feel good about their own sex and the opposite sex.

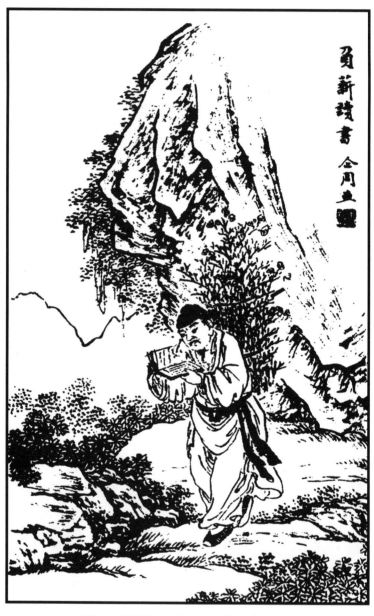

*Figure 16. By putting everything down on
paper I want to clarify my ideas.*

CHAPTER 9

More Notes from
a Dan-Tien Student

I am writing this book partly because I want to get better at using this incredible Dan-Tien concept. By putting everything down on paper I want to clarify my ideas and then share them with others. Here are some more notes from my diary:

October 18

Before I discovered Dan-Tien, part of my day was consumed by doubts, self-doubts, regrets, or resentments. While walking down the street, for example, I would wonder if I lived in the right place or associated with the right people. I would regret a wrong decision I made a year ago or envy someone who had something I did not have. I would blame some childhood experience or inherited flaw for my present problems. I would curse my parents, teachers, bosses, or other authorities when things went wrong in my life.

Now I know that it does not pay to make myself miserable with such thoughts. I focus instead on thoughts that feel good because they improve my life here and now. Then I get busy and do things that feel good in the Dan-Tien. I still think about the past now and then, and I realize that my life is influenced by all kinds of factors. But I do not allow myself to be tortured by painful trains of thought that lead nowhere. As soon as unpleasant feelings arise in my Dan-Tien, I wake up and get back on the happy road, where I am in tune with the universal life force. As soon as I feel that I am harmonizing with infinite intelligence, all the details of my life fall into place, and I know instinctively what to do next.

October 19

I like to live in tune with the "universal life force." This term is more all-inclusive than our Western concept of an almighty father god. By calling the life force a father, we exclude the motherly life force and degrade the female values. When people believe that only men are made in the image of God and the women are not, this distorts the whole fabric of society. It must create resentment in women and complacency in men.

The male-oriented Western mentality also looks down on the sexual and bodily functions, and on the Dan-Tien in particular. Pain in the body's center is ignored, and suffering is endured as normal. In most churches, the somber atmosphere serves as a constant reminder that suffering is a Christian virtue. In Islam it is customary to say: "Suffering is my greatest joy." Many Buddhists believe that life means suffering.

Taoism, on the other hand, has many aspects of a mother religion. Mother Nature does not torture her children. She guides them gently by sending them signals through the Dan-Tien. The original sin in Taoism is not sex, as in Christianity, but the habit of ignoring nature's signals, which is the root of all unhappiness, illness, and failure.

October 20

When I first explained all this to a friend yesterday, she asked if I had no ambitions or social conscience. Did I want to vegetate in my little world of navel contemplation? On the contrary, I said, I am now more aware than ever of other people's feelings and needs, simply because I understand myself better. And my life has become more adventurous and colorful since I discovered Dan-Tien. Above all, I have learned to enjoy every minute. My life now has meaning, it makes sense, and I have access to the life force.

My friend looked at me in disbelief. She had been unhappy for years, she said, although she had a wonderful family, a comfortable house, and a great deal of money. Every week she visited her psychiatrist who was now prescribing tranquilizers after years of analysis.

Then I mentioned that chemicals cannot solve problems, that they can only cover up the symptoms and allow the patient to continue his/her unnatural pattern of thinking and living. Freud, himself, had been a chain smoker, a cocaine addict, and a male chauvinist. Although he had some valuable insights over the years, he could not even solve his own problems.

My friend disagreed violently. My answers were too simple, she said. A few years ago I had thought so myself. Even now I can hardly believe that life can be so simple, rewarding, and enjoyable.

October 21

Last night I walked home from the train station. It was an enjoyable walk, and I looked forward to a special supper. I felt a pleasant rhythm and balance in my movements as I walked along.... But suddenly I sensed a change. There was a strain in my body, and I no longer felt the pleasant rhythm. I felt uncomfortable.

What had happened? Nothing around me had changed. But a negative emotion had crept in and upset my balance. I had remembered that a neighbor had borrowed my tool box with the promise to return it the next day. Now a week had passed and I had not heard from him.

I felt resentment. This man did not deserve my neighborly help! He had let me down! I despised unreliable people like him! I had good reason to get angry!

These were the thoughts and feelings that shot through my mind/body for a minute. But then I realized what was happening. It dawned on me that the anger was not really caused by my neighbor, but by my panicked reaction to a harmless event. I had allowed my mind to run wild, and I had lost touch with my Dan-Tien. The neighbor did not try to upset me. He had probably just forgotten the tool box.

The signal in my Dan-Tien had told me to find out what happened and to get the box back. It had not told me to get angry and to torture myself.

As soon as I became aware of this, my body relaxed, I enjoyed the rest of the walk, and my mind returned to pleasant and useful thoughts. I felt at home in my body, and the world looked fine once more.

Instead of fuming and hating the neighbor and myself, I dissolved the negative emotions and the physical strain in less than a minute, simply by following the messages of my Dan-Tien. Although the circumstances had not changed, the "problem" was gone, and I felt fine.

October 22

I often think of Lao Tzu, the Taoist philosopher who lived 2500 years ago. In his *Tao Te Ching* he said that "outside the Way everything is wrong." Whenever we lose touch with the Dan-Tien, everything we think and do is wrong. One sure sign of wrong thinking is the idea that life is not good enough or that we are not good enough. This is the idea that underlies all bad moods, depressions, misery, and unhappiness.

As soon as we find our way back into the Dan-Tien, all such thoughts and emotions disappear as if by magic. Suddenly the world looks good again, and the self-doubts are gone.

In one of his verses, Lao Tzu illustrates the importance of the center in all things:

Wheels are made of thirty spokes,
but their invisible essence lies in the central hub.
Bowls are made of clay,
but their usefulness lies in their hollow center.[1]

In the human mind/body the "invisible essence" is the Dan-Tien. The surface includes the skin, the five senses, the limbs, and the conscious mind. Yes, all our thinking is more or less superficial, it only scratches the surface. Even our profoundest thoughts can only grope for the "invisible essence." This includes the book I am writing now. No mere book can replace the real Dan-Tien experience, which is non-verbal.

October 23

Just now I felt depressed when I thought about the injustice of the legal system and the world in general. Countless innocent people are deprived of life, liberty, or property every day, while most criminals are never caught or convicted. What chance did an individual like me have in such a world? How could anyone enjoy life in such a corrupt society? I kept on finding more reasons for feeling miserable.

Then I remembered my motto: "When you feel miserable you have lost touch with Dan-Tien." Immediately I noticed my bent posture, superficial breathing and top-heavy behavior. After I got my body back to normal and shifted my mental focus down to the Dan-Tien, I felt relieved. Then I looked at my train of thought and decided to drop this preoccupation with one narrow subject that made me feel miserable. Why worry about things that I could not change? Why not think or do something useful and enjoyable? Why not focus on my blessings and opportunities?

Furthermore, could I claim to be such an angel who never hurt other people?

---

[1] Lao Tzu, *Tao Te Ching,* Translation into English mine, from a German source.

October 24

Something happens to my voice when I am centered in the Dan-Tien. It becomes deep and soothing, and people relax when they hear me talk. They are also more open to my ideas because they sense that my thoughts are in tune with life. Zen masters say that they can tell a student's progress by his voice. When the student is nervous and confused, his voice originates in the throat. When he calms down, the voice comes from the chest. But the truly centered person speaks from the center, from the bottom of the lungs.

October 27

Yesterday I felt resentment when I thought about my parents. This is, of course, the classic "childhood trauma" situation that bothers many people and provides fertile ground for psychoanalysis.

My first impulse was to accept this painful thought as a fact of life. We all feel justified in criticizing our parents now and then, don't we? But then I remembered my motto: "When a thought makes you feel bad in your Dan-Tien, you are on the wrong angle, you have lost touch with your Dan-Tien."

Here I had another opportunity to prove the effectiveness of the Dan-Tien concept. First I put myself into a more centered state of mind-body by becoming aware of posture, breathing, tension in the belly, etc. Then I thought about my parents again in this relaxed and "loving" frame of mind/body.

Now I saw a different picture. I suddenly realized that my parents probably did their best, that they also had been misunderstood in their childhood, and that they had their own problems.

Simply by looking at my "trauma" in a different way I had dissolved it, I had "burned" it in my Dan-Tien. I had neutralized the pain and was now ready to enjoy my present life again.

This approach differs radically from the conventional way of handling painful experiences. The accepted way is to either ignore or repress the problem, or to analyze and to relive it in the hope that it will go away. The Dan-Tien approach is more effective because it creates a good feeling first and then faces the pain in a relaxed way.

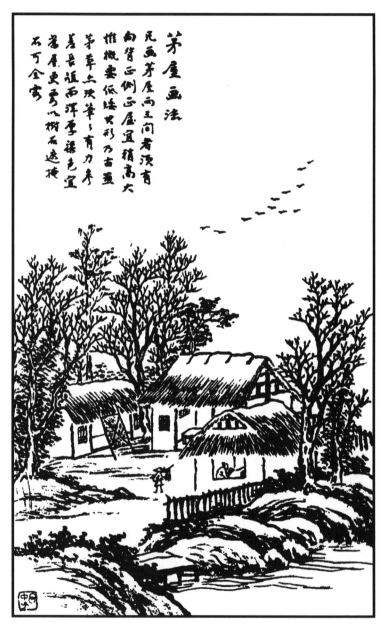

茅屋画法

凡画茅屋两三间者须宜
向背正侧正则屋宜稍高大
推概要低矮其形乃古逸
茅草之欢笔之有力方
若长短而洋季讲毛宜
苍屋虚秀以树石迤逗
石万全寄

Figure 17. The optimal location and shape of
gardens, buildings, windows, entrances.

At Home
in the World

Feng Shui, Shinto, and Taoism

To this day the Chinese have an intuitive feeling for the interrelationship between people and their natural surroundings. Especially in places like Hong Kong and Singapore they practice the ancient art of Feng Shui that has no equivalent in the West. A Feng Shui specialist is consulted before houses, buildings, or cities are planned. He measures the vibrations and magnetic lines, the lay of the land in relation to the course of the sun, the water flow on the surface and in subterranean veins. Although he uses computation tables, compasses, and other instruments, he also relies on his gut feelings, his Dan-Tien.

Thus he determines the optimal location and shape of gardens, paths, buildings, windows, entrances, and even cemetery plots. He makes sure that people live or die in harmony with nature, that they do not insult the spirits of the Earth, and that their descendants do likewise. Even most large commercial enterprises will not lease or build offices or factories before consulting a Feng Shui specialist who often charges substantial fees.

The Japanese also cultivate a close contact with nature. Their traditional Shinto religion is basically a joyful and spontaneous nature worship. Only in the last hundred years has it been given a militaristic slant. In ancient Japanese legend, Earth and the sea, the mountains and the forests, and nature in general, are born of the sacred union between male and female spirits, Izanagi and Izanami. The most important religious structure in Japan is the shrine at Ise, dedicated to the goddess Amaterasu. The Japanese emperor is said to be her descendant. This innocent faith in nature explains in part the incredible vitality and resilience of the Japanese people.

Underlying the Oriental concept of nature is the Chinese philosophy of Taoism and the Yin/Yang concept. This concept sees male and female, mind and body, culture and nature as complementing poles in a cosmic harmony. The poles balance and enhance each other, they are two sides of a coin. In the West, we tend to believe that one pole is "better" and must dominate the other. In our scriptures we are not admonished to harmonize with nature, but to dominate and exploit it. We are told to look upon nature as a resource, a threat, or a crude material that must be refined and civilized.

The essence of Taoist harmony with nature is condensed in the classic *Tao Te Ching* [The Right Way of Life]. The philosopher Lao Tzu wrote it 2500 years ago, on a mere eighty pages. According to this book the "eternal mother" is the root and source of everything. Her mysterious influence is invisible and has no name.

Lao Tzu describes the "right path of nature" (Tao), indicating that life is a journey, not a static arrangement. The Tao looks empty from the outside but is filled with inexhaustible energy. It is self-ordering and self-developing, self-balancing and self-healing, and ever-changing according to eternal laws. It is the base of all things in Heaven and on Earth, endlessly and effortlessly transforming the world. Its motherly force influences the course of events subtly and invisibly, without seeming to dominate.

To harmonize with this force should be our aim, according to ancient Chinese folk wisdom. Nothing is more important than our contact with nature. If we transgress against the laws of nature, we hurt ourselves and create confusion, illness, and chaos. But by living in tune with nature we are assured of health, abundance, and a long life.

Some Places Feel Good

In some places it is easier to feel good than in others. In certain houses or neighborhoods, for instance, we feel immediately at home, while in others we feel like strangers even after living there for a long time. In the same way we may feel attracted to certain landscapes and not to others. By listening to the signals from the Dan-Tien we can become more aware of the vibrations in each place. Although there may be times when we have to face unpleasant, ugly, or hostile environments, it is better to avoid such places when we have a choice.

Most of us live in homes or apartments that do not quite suit us. After a while we give up dreaming of the dream home and get used to reality. We stay where we are and make the best of the situation.

But are we really making the best of our home, such as it is? Have we tried everything and exhausted all possibilities? Have we succeeded in creating a comfortable "nest" for ourselves? Or are we just camping here in the hope that something better will turn up some day?

Quite often a place can be improved dramatically by making some simple but ingenious changes. What keeps us from making these changes is not so much the cost or a lack of interior decorating talent, but a lack of imagination and intuition. Our Dan-Tien can tell us how to make our house into a home, if we follow its subtle hints. Here is a list of ideas to stimulate the imagination:

- Add a touch of natural beauty through indoor plants or bunches of dry flowers. Place some of them on the floor, suspend others from the ceiling.
- Experiment with different types and colors of illumination. Lighting alone can make a room either cozy or cold.
- Create your own lampshades from baskets, rice paper or transparent cloth.

❧ Remove harsh ceiling lamps and neon lamps. Light from above usually creates a cold atmosphere, makes people look wrinkled and ugly.

❧ Create "his" and "hers" areas if space allows.

❧ Hide technical gadgets behind attractive curtains when they are not being used.

❧ Get some art reproductions or posters that you like. A good copy in a good frame can give a touch of beauty to a room.

❧ Your bathroom need not look cold and sterile. Cheerful shower curtains or floor mats can make all the difference.

❧ You may consider the Japanese custom of leaving your street shoes at the entrance, and using soft house shoes indoors. This is not only cleaner, but creates a more "homey" atmosphere.

❧ Most street clothes are not really comfortable or natural, and at home you may prefer to wear loose-fitting and colorful robes, for instance.

❧ If there is a garden, you can make it more interesting by adding a hill, a pond, or a corner for kitchen herbs.

❧ Colorful window curtains can add life to an otherwise drab room.

❧ Instead of hanging a still life painting on the wall, place a large bowl of colorful mixed fruit on the table.

❧ Use moveable partitions to change the atmosphere in a room according to changing needs.

❧ Keep in mind that round, organic forms and earthy colors make a place cozy, while straight forms and harsh colors do the opposite.

❧ While white bed linen is quite all right, you may enjoy sleeping between colors now and then.

❧ Reserve one shelf or wall for a collection of favorite items.

❧ If you are in a position to build your own home, use your imagination. Do not create a masterpiece of engineering, but a comfortable and beautiful nest that fits in with the natural surroundings.

At Home in Nature

It is easier to feel good in the Dan-Tien when we are surrounded by natural beauty. Our pagan ancestors enjoyed and worshiped nature. They often celebrated its beauty and majesty outdoors, near trees, springs, sacred ponds, creeks, caves, on hills and mountain tops. They lived in harmony with nature and treasured it.

But modern people think nothing of devastating their own natural environment, of polluting rivers and oceans, of letting vast forest areas die from air pollution, of destroying most of the tropical forests, and of sowing deadly atomic fall-out all over the globe.

The Western mind has lost touch with its own source. It looks upon nature as a challenge, an inconvenience, or a resource that must be exploited. Many of our religious buildings reflect this mentality—they resemble fortresses against nature. No plant or other living thing is allowed inside, and no window allows a view of the nature outside. Religious ceremonies are often performed indoors, in man-made, "civilized" surroundings, in a "spiritual" atmosphere set apart from nature.

Chinese and Japanese temples, on the other hand, blend in with nature. They are usually surrounded by beautifully landscaped gardens, with bamboo groves, fish ponds, flower beds, etc. Even the interior is often made to look like a garden, with large windows showing the beautiful nature outside. Such temples were made by people who lived in tune with their Dan-Tien, and anyone who enters them feels good inside.

The same mentality is reflected in Japanese and Chinese art. The great Chinese artists had an instinctive feeling for all natural phenomena. Their works usually reflect cyclical changes in the weather, the seasons, and the stages of growth. They picture aspects of the cosmic life force Chi and the subtle Yin/Yang balance in nature. According to a classic instruction manual for painters, the artist must first learn to become still in his center (Dan-Tien), to clarify his understanding, and to increase his wisdom.

Livable Communities

Our modern cities are masterpieces of engineering. But most of them lack natural charm, beauty and warmth, and people do not really feel at home in them. Our urban and suburban environments are straight, rectangular, efficient, and busy. They are also ugly, noisy, and polluted. They were not designed by people who lived in tune with their Dan-Tien. The people who must live there may get used to such conditions, but they will not really feel like human beings.

But is it possible to create livable communities in the machine age? Some architects in California came up with an answer that they called the "Pedestrian Pocket."[1] In effect they have re-invented the small town of yesteryear and added a modern touch. Instead of planning separate inner cities, industrial areas, and bedroom communities, as has been customary until now, they have designed integrated communities, where all daily needs are accessible in walking distance. A network of footpaths connects homes with schools and shops, so that children and elderly people can safely walk to their destinations.

A number of such pedestrian pockets are interconnected through a light rail system, and next to the rail lines run bicycle paths. Although people may still own and use automobiles, they will find it more convenient to do most errands by foot or to travel by light rail. A rail system is preferable to a bus system because it allows higher peak hour capacity.

Offices and light industry are located close to the rail stations, some of them near the community's center, so that workers can shop, eat in restaurants, or relax in the park during lunch hours. Each community is surrounded by nature and farm areas in walking distance. Air pollution, traffic congestion, and rush-hour traffic are no longer a problem. People stay healthier because they get more exercise through walking in fresh air. Children no longer need school buses, and the elderly no longer need

---

[1] Peter Calthorpe, "Pedestrian Pockets," *Whole Earth Review* (Spring 1988).

to stay at home for fear of being run over on busy streets. All parks and play areas are easily reached and unify the neighborhood, creating a community feeling that is missing in the customary suburban tract.

Dan-Tien and Television

Do people enjoy watching television? What a question! Of course they do! Why else would they spend hours in front of the TV set?

At least this is what they believe until they learn to listen to their Dan-Tien. Then they get the surprise of their life. They discover that they do not really feel good when they watch most of the programs. Perhaps they feel entertained, or stimulated, or excited. But unless they choose their programs very carefully, they will not really enjoy most of what they see.

How strange! People spend countless hours of their precious time in this way, in the mistaken belief that television brings them enjoyment. Millions even become addicted to this pursuit that actually reduces their well-being.

If they just switch on the set and watch whatever happens to be on at the moment, their chance of finding a program that really makes them "feel good" are slim indeed. But they usually keep watching anyway because they are entertained or because they think they have nothing better to do. Deep down, however, they know that they are wasting their time, and that the program will make them feel worse instead of better.

Then there is the fact that television tends to accentuate the sensational, the disturbing, and the abnormal. The screen shows the one person who has killed someone, for instance, and ignores the thousands of others who lead pleasant and normal lives. After watching such scenes all day, the viewer gets the impression that all human beings are more or less crazy.

The advertising messages between programs are futhermore designed to make people feel dissatisfied. Anyone who does not have the advertised product or service is pictured as ignorant or inferior. The "messages from our sponsor" are by their very nature one-sided, misleading, and insincere, with few exceptions. Some TV programs are excellent, of course—if we can find them! A few are really informative and enjoyable, and we would not want to miss them. The trouble with television is that we usually end up watching the wrong programs. Too often we stuff ourselves with images and information that do not really concern us and merely disturb our peace of mind.

What Music Does to Us

Of course we like music—everybody does! Music can be exhilarating, exciting, inspiring, or soothing. But it can also get on our nerves and decrease our mental and physical well-being.

As we become more aware of the Dan-Tien, we appreciate each piece of music for what it really does to us. Our tastes become more selective and discriminating. We realize that we enjoy certain melodies because they make us feel good—not just because they happen to be in fashion or because others like them.

The music of J. S. Bach, for instance, is considered a model of musical perfection by many. But when we hear it and listen also to the Dan-Tien, we may notice a certain rigid monotony in it that we may or may not like.

Modern 12-tone music is undoubtedly interesting and novel, but does it really make us feel good? A composer of modern music, Arnold Schoenberg, had the ambition to write scores for Hollywood films. He succeeded several times, and each time his music was chosen as a background for horror movies.

Music from the Islamic countries sounds intriguingly exotic, but we can sense a sad quality about it, as if it were performed by tortured souls. The word *Islam* means submission, incidentally, and the music is intended to get us into a submissive mood.

Is hard rock music really an expression of youthful exuberance? Researchers like Dr. John Diamond[2] have found that the rock rhythm produces stress and tension in the body because it is antagonistic to the natural heartbeat. A certain destructive men-

---

[2] See John Diamond, *Your Body Doesn't Lie* (New York: Warner, 1989).

tality can also be detected in the rock lyrics and CD covers. Experiments with plants have shown that rock music tends to harm or kill them, while they thrive with folk music, Viennese waltzes, the Beatles, or Baroque music. We can guess what the exposure to this music does to children and others who are emotionally vulnerable.

But there are plenty of other types of music that make us feel good—and sometimes we feel even better when we enjoy silence. We do not have to suffer helplessly from unpleasant or destructive vibrations. Our Dan-Tien can tell us what is good for us at any given time.

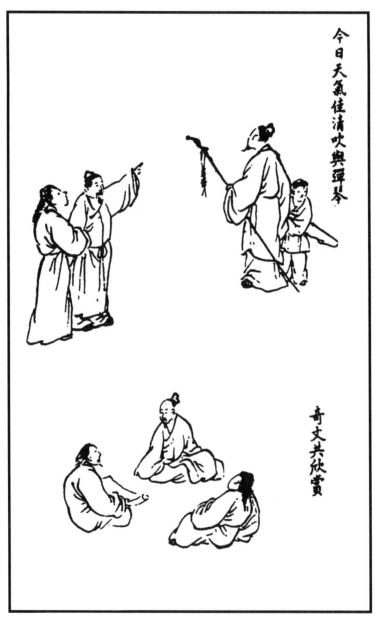

Figure 18. A kind attitude toward others and yourself.

Enjoyable
Relationships

In Tune with Others and Yourself

Being centered in the Dan-Tien means having a kind attitude toward others and yourself. You see something worthwhile in almost everybody, and you look for the good in each situation. At the same time you see yourself as worthwhile and likable, and you harmonize with human nature in general. To "love your neighbor" is not a duty or a moral precept, but a spontaneous need. Only people who ignore their Dan-Tien will try to be loving and altruistic from a sense of duty, moral obligation, or bad conscience.

When you are more aware of your own feelings, you also become aware of other people's feelings. When you feel good about yourself, most of your relationships also become pleasant, and you know how to handle unpleasant ones. As others sense your inner harmony by your facial expression and other non-verbal messages, they tend to react in kind, even before you have said a word.

People like to be loved, appreciated, and accepted, and they fear criticism. If you criticize them, they close up, fight back, or

85

do the opposite of what you want them to do. They obviously think that what they are doing is right, otherwise they would not do it. Even the worst criminals are usually convinced that their actions are justified. They have explanations and rationalizations for everything they do.

Instead of telling people that they are wrong, it is normally better to ignore their faults and to talk about their good points. Instead of trying to teach them, we can set a constructive example by living in tune with our Dan-Tien. Before people can drop their negative old habits, they have to be convinced that there is a better solution waiting for them.

All this also applies to the way we treat ourselves, of course. Self-criticism or self-contempt do more harm than good. It is better to build on our successes and to compliment ourselves at each step forward.

Love Relationships

Love is nice, and to love and be loved feels good. Men and women are simply made for each other; they need and complement each other. But because they have differing functions, they see life from slightly different angles, and this can lead to occasional frictions and misunderstandings.

Men are more Yang and women are more Yin, and when they love each other they experience cosmic union. When the two sexes harmonize, they experience the harmony of all aspects of the Yin/Yang polarity: between thoughts and feelings, mind and body, conscious and unconscious mind, spirit and matter, heaven and earth, etc.

When there is trust between man and woman, occasional disagreements will not harm the relationship. But before the two can feel good about each other, they have to feel good about themselves individually. If one partner secretly despises him/herself, he/she will try to undermine the self-confidence of the other, through nagging or negative remarks.

People who truly love each other also love each other's bodies, and they feel at home in their own bodies. The physical attraction is there from the moment they first meet. As soon as the first spark of sexuality is ignited, the mutual journey has begun. When both partners are aware of the duality of creation, they can experience it in each other and begin to merge in mind and body. No specific act in this process is more important than any other. Holding hands, the first kiss, a picnic in the park, or a swim in the lake bring as much joy as the actual sexual act. With experienced lovers the intercourse is merely another incident in the continuing art of love.

The amateurish preoccupation with intercourse is most prevalent in Western societies, where the goal is considered more important than the journey, where love turns into a hectic race to reach the all-important orgasm. This mentality brings more frustration than joy because it means that people spend 99.9 percent of their lives yearning, scheming, and hoping for a few minutes of intercourse. They miss all the flowers and the beauty along the way.

All this happens when people lose touch with their feelings and their Dan-Tien. By finding their center again they can enjoy every minute and all aspects of their love relationship in a continuous honeymoon.

It Feels Good to be Loved and Needed

Most of our thoughts and actions involve other people, although we may seldom be aware of this. We eat food that is produced by others, we wear clothes that others have made, we live in homes that others have built. Almost everything we know and believe has been created by the minds of others, and we even use a language that has been passed on to us.

But how we experience this social environment is determined by our own condition. The most favorable social environment cannot do anything for us if we do not enjoy inner harmony, if we do not live in tune with our Dan-Tien. As long as we cannot enjoy our own company, we cannot really enjoy the company of others. We may use others to distract and entertain ourselves, but in the end all relationships will disappoint us. Just as we use others, we get the feeling that others use us.

Yet we are social animals, and we like to be loved and needed. What happens when human beings grow up without the benefit of a social network? Several cases are known of babies who were abandoned in the woods and raised by wild animals. In India, two sisters grew up as members of a pack of wolves. When they were discovered by villagers, they were about 10 years old. They walked on hands and feet and communicated by howling like wolves. For food they accepted only raw meat, which they could smell from a distance of 50 yards, and they never got used to cooked food. Efforts to teach them how to walk normally and to speak even a few words were in vain.

This and other examples show how thoroughly each human being is molded by the social environment. It is hard to imagine the true extent of all social influences. The human being as we know it simply would not exist without them.

But although the social influence is strong, there is plenty of room for individual freedom. There is actually no contradiction between our social and our private interests. Healthy societies manage to create a harmony or synergy between private and public interests, so that the aspirations of the individual coincide normally with those of the community. In the less harmonious societies both parties see each other as a threat or an enemy. This conflict can only be resolved when people gradually learn to live in tune with their Dan-Tien.

The Harmonious Community

Ruth Benedict coined the word "synergy" to describe the state of harmony between individual and communal drives. In her anthropological studies of American Indians and South Sea Island tribes she discovered many examples of good and bad synergy. On the west coast of Canada she came upon a tribe that did not know private property because everything was shared. Among the Zuñis of New Mexico it is considered bad manners to win in competitive events. In other tribes property was tolerated, but wealthy people were despised because they kept everything for themselves.[1]

Benedict came to the conclusion that modern American society is not very synergetic, and that the prevailing culture makes people too competitive and acquisitive. It rewards greed and egotism, and it degrades people who enjoy sharing and living simply. The great American dream is to become a millionaire, and most American men consider themselves failures when they do not reach this goal. The means by which the money is acquired are almost irrelevant, even if they are socially destructive or on the verge of criminality.

Lao Tzu's Ideal Community

Lao Tzu, the great Taoist philosopher, described an ideal social order in his famous *Tao Te Ching*. He explained that this order must be based on the natural order of the universe, that it must harmonize with Tao, the Way of Nature. The cosmos is self-developing, self-ordering, and ever-changing. It is the root of all things in Heaven and on Earth, endlessly transforming the world. Its motherly qualities influence the course of events subtly and humbly, without seeming to dominate.

To harmonize with this force should be our aim. People who interfere with the natural order only hurt themselves and create chaos. We feel strong through contact with the Tao, by subduing the ego and flowing with the current of nature. To crave power, prestige, or possessions is foolish because these things make us dependent on the mercy of others, they reduce our sense of freedom.

People have an inborn desire to be good and moral. These qualities are brought out by a simple and innocent life under wise leadership. Good rulers subtly and invisibly influence society by paying attention to developments in their beginning stages rather than using force later. Any attempt to create order by strict laws, police action, or war only brings on more chaos and frus-

---

[1] Ruth Benedict, *Patterns of Culture* (Boston: Houghton Mifflin, 1989).

tration. When society harmonizes with the Tao, the interests of individuals coincide with those of society. It is only the clumsy leaders who formulate policies that conflict with human nature or who set a bad example by leading extravagant and ostentatious lives.

Leaders should remember that they evolved from the people, that they owe their position to the people, and that they are a product of the society that they are trying to lead. They should be aware of this mutual dependence and pay attention to the grass roots. Large problems are usually the result of subtle conflicts that were neglected in the past. Subtle and adaptable leaders become great because they pay attention to details, while strong and aggressive leaders provoke conflicts and accidents. The wealth of society should be distributed fairly evenly, so that people have no reason to become envious, and there is no temptation to steal. In his *Tao Te Ching,* Lao Tzu said:

> The Tao is eternal and nameless.
> Its nature is simple yet unchanging.
> If rulers would follow it,
> the people would gladly follow them in turn.
> heaven and earth would unite,
> sweet dew would fall on everything,
> and harmony would reign everywhere.
> But when the mind starts cutting the world apart,
> it is time to stop it.
> To know when to stop means to avoid danger.
> Only by following the Tao can the many streams
> flow together in a river of harmony.[2]

---

[2] Lao Tzu, *Tao Te Ching,* D. C. Lau, trans. (London: Penguin, 1963), Verse 32.

CHAPTER 12

The Answer is Closer than We Think

Pleasant and Unpleasant Feelings

Life is really quite simple. There are two types of feelings and thoughts: those that feel good in the Dan-Tien and those that do not. When we feel good, most of our thoughts are useful, constructive, and healing. When we do not feel good, most of our thoughts are useless, destructive, accident-prone, and unhealthy. Here is a basic list:

Feeling Good	**Not Feeling Good**
Feeling at home in your body.	Feeling ill at ease in your body.
Enjoying the body functions.	Despising the body functions.
Enjoying the Here and Now.	Worrying about the past, future, other places.
Enjoying everyday projects and challenges.	Doing things absent-mindedly, grudgingly.
Planning and picturing a radiant future.	Nervous confusion, lack of realistic planning.

91

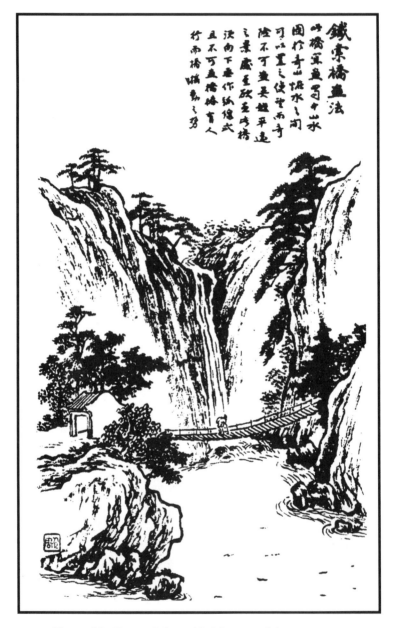

Figure 19. Harmonizing with Nature and human nature.

Being creative, self-reliant, taking the initiative.	Feeling at the mercy of past and future, or people or fate in general.
Being kind to others and yourself.	Criticizing others and yourself.
Minding your own business.	Worrying about other people's business.
Harmonizing with nature and human nature.	Being out of tune with nature and human nature.
Benefiting from past experiences, learning from mistakes.	Regretting and lamenting the past, feeling guilty and helpless.
Feeling close to a cosmic source or infinite intelligence.	Feeling lost in a senseless, meaningless universe.
Feeling grateful to be alive, finding life rich and worthwhile.	Feeling that life is not good enough, you are not good enough.
Feeling good all over, in every limb, muscle, and nerve.	Feeling full of tension, anger, self-pity, envy, resentment, etc.

Whenever we are not centered in the Dan-Tien, we experience life as described in the right column above. But as soon as we begin to live in tune with the Dan-Tien, we enjoy life more and more in the ways described in the left column.

The Wandering Mind

A famous Zen master had reached the highest level of consciousness. When asked how he occupied his mind during the day, he replied: "When eating I eat, when fetching water I fetch water, and when I go to bed I sleep."

His mind was centered and collected, it was involved only with the thing he was doing at the moment. He did not waste his time with useless, aimless thinking.

The opposite is true of the person who is not centered in his Dan-Tien. If we could read his or her mind in the course of a day, we would find his or her mind flitting about nervously. The day might start like this:

7:43 A.M. I sit down at the breakfast table, look out the window, and notice the cloudy sky...think I may get wet on the way to work...just like my neighbor Mike did yesterday...Mike's wife looks different lately...

7:44 She uses make-up...maybe she has a lover on the side...I'll pour a cup of coffee now...Columbian coffee probably...they still grow coffee there, although cocaine is more profitable... people are getting into drugs more and more...and the world is getting uglier...but I will just have to put up with it...

7:45 I am a victim of this greedy and corrupt system...now shall I put jelly or marmalade on my toast?...the toast is burned...these toasters never work properly...just like my car... I spend 26 percent of my income on this car and get nothing but trouble...

7:46 Now there is someone parking his car right in front of my house...why do they always park here?...the world is getting more crowded every day...just imagine what it will be like in a hundred years...it is already ten to eight...I have to go...didn't even have time to enjoy my breakfast...now it is raining...what a miserable day...hope this boss isn't grumpy today . . .

And so it goes. Minute after minute the mind wanders about without aim or reason. It is a helpless victim of chance events, painful memories, and worries. It is busy with irrelevant thoughts and negative emotions that just happen to pop up. It gets side-tracked by useless mental movies. Only now and then does the mind get down to the business of the moment, of focusing joyfully on present concerns. Many people can feel really good only during emergencies or under pressure when they have something definite to do, when there is no time for aimless thinking.

How can we avoid all this "busy-thinking" and use our mind sensibly and constructively? By finding our center and living in tune with Dan-Tien. When we become aware of the signals from the center, we can stop the painful, aimless thinking and focus on relevant things that make us feel good.

How Do You Feel?

How do you feel right now? Set aside a quiet minute to become aware of your physical self. Do you feel good in your body? In your legs? Around your neck and shoulders? Around your throat? And in the stomach area? Do you feel really good everywhere? Can you say that you really feel "at home in your body"? Or do you detect a slight tension here, a strange sensation there, a heavy feeling all over, a tight feeling, or a dull pain somewhere?

If you have never done anything like this before, or if you have been taught to ignore your feelings, you may feel little or nothing at first. The sensitivity you had as a child may have been lost, especially in school and other authoritarian institutions.

Even if you are aware of these body sensations, you may dismiss them as meaningless or irrelevant. "There is always some little friction here or there," you may say, "and I am not going to worry about this. My body is an imperfect machine with its little kinks, and the main thing is that I keep it under control."

Your body is in fact highly intelligent. Everything it does has a meaning. When it sends out unpleasant sensations, it is sending you a message, a warning signal. It tells you that you are thinking or doing something that is useless or harmful.

You can compare your body to an airplane. Whenever there is a fault in the machine or the way it flies, little warning lights start flashing. They ask you to pay attention and to correct the problem.

Your body is full of such "warning lights," your Dan-Tien being the central alarm point. When you feel really good all over, and especially in your center, you have been given the green light. This pleasant feeling tells you in effect: "Go ahead, all is well. Whatever you are thinking or doing at the moment is just what the present situation calls for." You are on the radar beam, so to speak, and you can relax in the sure knowledge that you are on the right track.

Feel Your Way

Suppose you suddenly feel uncomfortable while reading this book. You detect an unpleasant feeling in the belly area. It is nothing serious or alarming, but still a warning signal, a little flashing red light. What does it tell you? The message is clear: you are somehow on the wrong track.

Now you want to get back to normal, you want to feel good all over again. You don't want to force yourself to read with the tension in your Dan-Tien. You want to enjoy this book. Or perhaps you want to put the book aside and do something more important.

But what exactly should you do to get rid of the unpleasant sensation and the negative thoughts or emotions that come with it? *The answer is always:* Feel your way until it feels good again.

Start by checking your physical condition. Are you sitting in a comfortable and balanced posture? Have you been sitting too long, should you get up and stretch, or take a short walk? Has your breathing been superficial? Did you eat too little or too much? Do you feel hot or cold?

Quite often the whole "problem" can be solved on this level, without any need to go further into your emotions or thoughts. Your posture can also affect the way you feel.

If, after checking all bodily aspects, your Dan-Tien still feels funny, you can ask yourself questions like: "Do I feel resentment or anger toward something or somebody at this moment? Is my thinking distorted by worry or fear right now? Am I plagued by feelings of guilt, self-pity, or regret?"

Remember that all such distorted thoughts and feelings will seem perfectly "logical" and "necessary" to you while you are in this negative state. Do not trust your intellect now, trust your

Dan-Tien. As long as you feel funny in your Dan-Tien, this shows with absolute certainty that you are on the wrong track. On this route you will not get anywhere, and you will waste your time and energy. You must find the route that feels good.

Keep feeling your way until you come upon a thought or activity that feels good. Keep digging until you find a gold mine of joy. You will find it in the most unexpected direction. You can do all this in a matter of minutes or even seconds.

Dan-Tien is Different

By probing in different directions in this way you have found the touchy point and removed it. From the way you feel good again you know that your thoughts and emotions are now back on the right track. Whatever you think or do in this happy state makes sense, it is useful, meaningful, and constructive. Once more you feel confident in your ability to solve problems and to get results in your daily life. You also know that you will enjoy almost every minute.

Note the difference between the Dan-Tien approach used here and the route that is usually followed. Normally you would have ignored your body sensations, and thus you would have remained unaware of your negative state. You would have let yourself wallow in any negative (unhappy) thoughts and emotions that came along. You would have been tempted to dig yourself deeper into far-fetched or useless theories, speculations, unpleasant memories, mental movies, worries, regrets, resentments, etc. This you would have called "dealing with the problem and explaining its causes."

This is also the route followed by most psychotherapists, a never-ending route that brings occasional "insights" but no real solutions, even after years of expensive treatment. Since most therapists use this approach in their own lives, underneath the professional veneer they are usually just as unhappy and mixed up as their patients. Freud, himself, was a chain smoker, a cocaine addict, and a male chauvinist, which tells us something about his prevailing state of mind.

Our Normal and Natural Condition

By centering the Chi energy in the Dan-Tien, we dissolve negative emotions as soon as they crop up. In this way we are liberated, for all practical purposes, from their destructive influences, and we can enjoy life as free and happy persons. In this state of mental and physical well-being we are in tune with the Self, we are in our normal and natural condition. Anything less than that would really be "subnormal" and below our standards. Others may accept negative states as normal, but for us they are unacceptable.

But as we become more aware of our Dan-Tien in the coming days and weeks, we will discover to our surprise that we slip into the negative state quite often. During an average day this may happen dozens of times, and each time we will tend to get entangled in a string of useless thoughts.

Gradually we will learn to avoid these traps or to get out of them in a hurry. We will enjoy our normal happy state for longer and longer periods, with very few interruptions. Life becomes a pleasant journey, and we experience inner harmony, a delight of being alive, and kindness toward others and ourselves. We become aware of the underlying harmony that was there all the time but had been crowded out by inner and outer stress. By thus weeding our garden we can let the flowers bloom again.

The quality of our life really depends on the quality of our feelings about ourselves and the world at any given moment. Our world looks unpleasant or ugly whenever we lose touch with our Dan-Tien. The same world can suddenly be full of love and sunshine when we are centered again.

If inner friction is harmful, does this mean that we should be relaxed at all times? Not really. Relaxing is a good idea when we have been too tense, but it is not a cure-all. Total relaxation would be a form of sleep or death. What we really want is a subtle state of "being here and now" or "restful alertness." We can reach and maintain this state only when we are centered in our Dan-Tien.

Poor Substitutes for Dan-Tien

Usually without knowing it, people living in the modern world are deprived of the primal elementary pleasure that wild animals and humans living close to nature take for granted every day. They are caught in a state of unease that disturbs and undermines the basic mind/body processes that are meant to keep them happy and healthy. They are no longer in touch with their center of joy and vitality, their Dan-Tien.

People who feel thus deprived will search for fulfillment in other ways. Many will try to keep busy making more and more money or acquiring more and more gadgets and status symbols. Others will accumulate titles, diplomas, medals, honors, fame, and power. A few will seek consolation in the fanatical pursuit of spiritual or intellectual endeavors. Many will try to soothe the inner pain with alcohol, through over-eating, or by desperately seeking company of any kind. Some will depend on soothing drugs to relieve the inner tension, or they will use mind-expanding drugs to break out of their mental cages.

Yet others will try to drown out the inner friction with continuous television watching, ear-shattering music, or noisy motor vehicles. Some will even plunge headfirst into dangerous, life-threatening adventures, merely to divert the attention from the inner pain for a while.

Such pursuits could also be beneficial if used in moderation, of course. But to the people who have lost touch with their Dan-Tien, these activities become irrational attempts to make up for the missing harmony. Millions of people spend much of their time, money, and energy chasing after illusory goals in this way. Large segments of the economy exist mainly or entirely to cater to their misguided search for inner contentment. Advertisers cunningly exploit people's cravings by promising never-ending happiness to the buyer of this or that product, even if the product is, in fact, useless or harmful.

Is this discontent necessary? Is it the price we have to pay for the blessings of civilization, as Sigmund Freud and others have suggested? Or does it in fact indicate that there is something fundamentally wrong with our civilization? Those who know the secret of Dan-Tien have discovered a better solution.

Dan-Tien: Better than Biofeedback

Sometimes the body may seem like a crude mechanism that must be controlled and disciplined by the mind. Yet nothing could be further from the truth. The body is incredibly subtle and complex, and it has its own wisdom. It actually bristles with millions of tiny transmitters and receivers and is guided by a sophisticated mind of its own.

This is what biologist Barbara Brown found when she used complex electronic equipment to listen in to the body.[1] Her experiments showed that mind and body are really two sides of a coin. All our thoughts affect the body in some way, and all body processes influence our thoughts and emotions in turn. She began to use the term "mind-body" to describe the human organism.

In one experiment she demonstrated this with the help of toy trains and flashing lights. By connecting her equipment to the skin of a test person, she caused lights to flash and toy trains to start up whenever the person's brain was calm and centered and produced alpha waves. After some weeks of training the person then learned to produce this state of mind at will. Brown coined the word "biofeedback" to describe this learning process.

After years of research Brown came to the conclusion that the body is usually more wise than the mind, that its reactions tend to be more in tune with life. When there is a conflict between mind and body, the mind does more harm than good when it forces the body to obey.

In our Western culture we are taught to assume that the mind is always right. We like to impose discipline and authoritarian

---

[1] Interested readers may want to explore Barbara B. Brown's, *New Mind, New Body* (New York: Harper & Row, 1974).

rule on the body. When the body malfunctions or revolts, we again blame it for causing trouble and we use stronger methods to "keep it under control."

This unhappy relationship then leads to nervous problems, psychosomatic illness and various diseases. Barbara Brown believes that most of our modern psychological, medical, and even social problems could be prevented if we listened to our bodies more often. A growing number of researchers in different fields agree with her. More and more doctors realize that mental and physical health go hand in hand, and that a good healer must look at the whole person rather than focus on the diseased part only. More and more people become body-conscious and use words like "psychosomatic" which simply means "mind/body."

But although the biofeedback experiments were a step in the right direction, they did not fulfill their initial promise. It turned out that good equipment is not only expensive but also difficult to operate. The method is therefore not suited for everyday use by an untrained person.

The ideal biofeedback device exists however. It is in fact built into the large bio-computer that we call the human body. The subtlety and complexity of this built-in feedback device exceeds anything that electronic science could invent. We can perceive it and make use of it through the Dan-Tien. Only now are we discovering how effective and useful this device is. We are beginning to realize that life can be meaningful, rewarding, beautiful, and enjoyable only when we live in tune with the Dan-Tien.

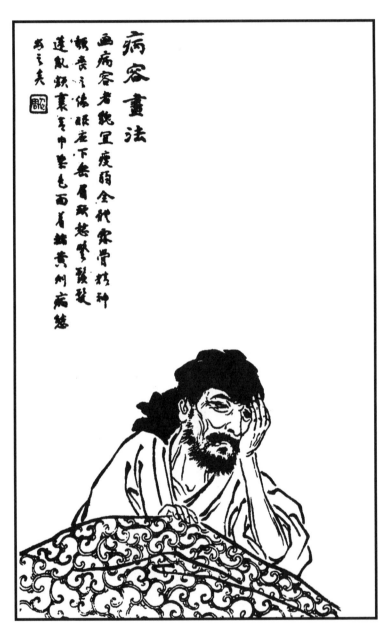

*Figure 20. Yet such problems of the past
can be solved quickly and easily.*

CHAPTER 13

Getting into
the Dan-Tien Habit

Problems of the Past

Many people feel weighed down by unhappy memories. Psycho-analysts of the Freudian school explain most problems through childhood traumas. The Hindus in India feel weighed down by their sins in previous incarnations. Two hundred million Indians are known as "Untouchables." They have supposedly committed awful crimes in their previous lives, and must therefore perform only the dirtiest work. In Western countries millions of people feel equally condemned to endure a life of relative unhappiness and years of costly psychoanalysis because of supposed or suspected childhood traumas.

Yet such problems of the past can be solved quickly and easily. They disappear automatically when we live in tune with the Dan-Tien. Simply by dissolving the negative emotions that relate to these past experiences, we can turn traumas into harmless memories.

We may, for instance, resent or hate a person who hurt us many years ago. Or we may feel sorry for ourselves because we believe that we have been mistreated by relatives, employers, teachers, authorities, or by fate in general. How can we possibly solve such problems when the damage has long been done? Simply by relating to the past in a new way.

The picture of our past, as we see it, is not objective but highly subjective. We are perfectly capable of creating a biased and partly fictitious picture of the past (or future) that supports and justifies our present attitude of self-pity and resentment. Even Freud admitted this in his later works. It is only too human to blame the past (about which we can do nothing) for a present problem about which we *can* do something.

The focal point of our life is not our past or our future, but the present moment. It is what we do *now* that counts. Our life is right as long as our *current* attitude toward present, past, and future is right. Simply by "sensing the Dan-Tien" we can find out whether our picture of the past feels right or not. By feeling our way we can soon arrive at a picture of our past that feels good because it does justice to all involved.

Imaginary Traumas

By thus centering our Chi energy in the Dan-Tien, we can dissolve painful memories. Even childhood traumas that have bothered, depressed, or limited us for years can be transcended in this way, often in a matter of minutes.

But this magic works both ways, and we can actually "create" childhood traumas just as fast as we can dissolve them. We have done this unintentionally many times and have suffered the consequences. Whenever we are tense and confused, past problems multiply or get worse. All aspects of our past tend to look gloomy as soon as we lose touch with our body and our Dan-Tien.

This is so because we invariably project our present feelings into our picture of the past (or future). For example, if we feel inferior at this very moment, we will tend to remember occasions in our past when we failed at something. If we now feel lucky, on the other hand, we tend to remember occasions when we were lucky.

To convince yourself of this, you can make a simple experiment. Some day when you feel a little depressed, accentuate this feeling by bending your posture, breathing in a hectic way and staring at things with tense eyes. Stretch your head forward and breathe nervously from the shoulders for some time. Force your body into uncomfortable and unnatural positions while you walk, sit, or stand.

Soon you will notice a change in the way you feel and think. When you now think about your past and your childhood, unpleasant mental associations will tend to come up. Pictures of unhappy events and traumatic experiences may appear. One or two "traumas" may stand out in your imagination, and you may dramatize and magnify them. Then you may conclude that here lies the root of your present problems.

You have in fact created a myth, a mixture of fact and fantasy that enables you to blame present problems on supposed past problems. Suddenly you feel like the helpless victim of people or of fate.

This example illustrates that it is not so much our past that shapes our life, but our present state of mind/body. By living in tune with our Dan-Tien, we can get into the habit of feeling good about present, past, and future.

Finding the Right Angle

When it starts to rain while we are walking in the country, and we forgot to take our raincoat, we've got a problem. When we feel miserable because of a childhood trauma or an accident, that is also a problem. And when we tell people that our car has just been stolen, that our wife/husband has left us, or that we have been fired, they will say: "You've got a problem there." What do all these examples have in common? They all make us feel unhappy.

The emphasis here is on the word "feel." Our feelings are highly individual and subjective. What bothers other people may not be a problem to us and vice versa. To be aware of this fact alone can help us solve many a problem, big or small. For example, if someone says: "This weather is terrible," we may be tempted to feel "under the weather" too, even though the weather does not really bother us at all.

Unhappy feelings can disappear within minutes or even seconds when we approach the problem from the right angle. The problem then disappears also because it is no longer associated with unhappy feelings. Objectively speaking "the problem" may still be there, but we no longer experience it as such. We are no longer dominated or irritated by it. We know that we can handle it and that we are in control. Strictly speaking it was not the problem that bothered us, but our unhappy mental associations.

This applies to all problems, regardless of type or size, and regardless of time or location. It does not matter whether we perceive the problem in our past or in a far-away place. We can still solve it in a matter of minutes, simply by finding our center again. This is especially true of normal everyday problems, and it is a great help even in more tragic situations.

How do we know which is the right approach and the suitable course of action? By feeling our way. Our Dan-Tien will let us know when we are on the right track again. Suddenly we feel good about ourselves and our world.

Even money problems become more manageable when we approach them in this way. Money in itself is neither good nor bad, but our present attitude toward money may be. Do we feel good about the way we handle money—the way we earn it and the way we spend it? Or do we have mixed feelings and negative emotions regarding this important subject? Money is really a form of life energy that flows between us and others. When this flow makes us feel good in our Dan-Tien, we know that we are on the right track.

The Habit of Enjoying Every Minute

When we get into the habit of enjoying life from minute to minute, we are as close to lasting happiness and fulfillment as a human being can ever be. Life, after all, is nothing but a succession of minutes, and we are always "here and now."

The past is gone, and the future exists only in our imagination. To regret the past and to worry about the future is a waste of time and energy, and it only makes us feel unhappy. But to do something worthwhile here and now is fun, and this includes making plans for the future and learning from the past. Living in the here and now means living the good life, while the habit of straying from the here and now is the beginning of all problems, suffering, and illness.

By living in tune with the Dan-Tien, we not only solve problems, but we can prevent them in the first place. As we go through the day, almost every second brings subtle shifts and changes. As we become more and more aware of our Dan-Tien, we detect the little guiding hints from our center, step by step.

> One minute you wonder if it would be wise to make an important telephone call now, or would it be better to go in person?
>
> A few seconds later you remember an unpleasant episode. Is there something you can do about it, or is it better to forget it?
>
> Now you want to sit down in the dining room, or would it be nicer in the garden?
>
> A little later you get ready for your shopping, or would you really prefer to see the neighbor first?
>
> Thirty seconds later you are talking to the neighbor. Will you talk about the weather and the garden? Or would you want to talk about something that is closer to the neighbor's heart? And so on.

All such minute-to-minute shifts are continuously taking place, and we hardly notice them. Yet these are the precious minutes of which 99 percent of our life is made up. If we do not feel good inside during most of these minutes, then we simply do not feel good about our whole life. We may say that we feel okay and are happy now and then. But deep down we know that we feel frustrated most of the time. Perhaps we still have some hopes for the future. But even the future is bound to disappoint us if we do not get into the habit of enjoying every minute.

Gradually, over the weeks and months, we can learn to enjoy the present moment. After a while we will notice to our surprise how our life has changed. We may also notice that others often get caught up in unhappy moods and negative emotions. They are still at the stage where we were before we learned the secret of Dan-Tien.

The Practical Angle

Each unpleasant sensation in the Dan-Tien is accompanied by negative emotions and useless thoughts. All three are interconnected. They arise together, and they also disappear together. Here lies the key to the solution of any problem. We can start by:

A) doing something about our thoughts,
B) or by becoming aware of our emotions,
C) or by rebalancing our body, posture, breathing, or movements.

We can shift from one area to another, in a continuous process, until the unpleasant sensation in the Dan-Tien disappears.

Common sense will usually tell us where to begin. Perhaps we have been sitting in a slumping position for hours, and we feel better as soon as we get up and stretch. Perhaps we detect a negative emotion such as self-pity or resentment, and we feel better as soon as we admit this to ourselves and do something about it. Or perhaps we notice that we have been dominated by useless thoughts or mental movies, and we feel better as soon as we switch to more important thoughts and begin to put them into action. Any angle is worth trying, as long as it makes us feel good in the Dan-Tien again. With some creative imagination we can figure out just what our real needs are at the moment.

Psychologists may argue forever over the question of what is more important: the body, the mind, or the emotions. Did the chicken come first, or the egg, or the nest, or indeed the rooster? But in practice it really makes no difference, and we may just as well say that they all came into being at the same time. Any approach will do, as long as it makes us feel good in the Dan-Tien.

Negative Thoughts

Negative (unhappy) thoughts and emotions have little or nothing to offer. We cannot learn anything from them. Basically it would be all right to dwell on them, except that we have more important things to do. We do not want to ignore or suppress them, we just have no time for them.

If we do think about them occasionally, we find that they are all interconnected. They are all joined together at the root, like the tentacles of an octopus. When we start to pull at one leg, we gradually end up with all the other legs, too. If we are dominated by a feeling of resentment, for instance, there will also be an underlying sense of:

Self-pity, because we feel mistreated by someone or by fate.

Hate, because we want to get even with someone.

Envy, because we feel that other people have more than they deserve, that we deserve what they have.

Guilt, because we secretly hope or plan for the misfortune of others.

Regret, because we feel that we should have done something about this sooner and that we have made other mistakes.

Anger, because we feel that some people have misunderstood or mistreated us, even in our childhood.

The more we dig into any of these items, the more we get entangled with the whole octopus. More unhappy memories emerge and more miserable feelings about ourselves and the world in general. This is the fertile ground on which some therapists earn their lucrative incomes. This is the main reason why they encourage their patients to talk and talk about their problems, and to dwell on their mistakes and traumatic experiences.

Most psychological theories are in fact based on the observation of mental patients and other disturbed people. These people are suffering from "complexes" of problems—they are at the mercy of the whole octopus. As a result most psychologists emphasize the neurotic aspects of human nature. A notable exception is the "humanistic" psychology of Abraham Maslow, who based his findings not on mental patients, but on the study of "normal" and successful people. He is well-known for his "hierarchy of human needs" and his studies of self-realization and peak experiences. He found that human beings are by nature kind and eager to help each other, that they are creative and open to divine inspiration, and that they have many other desirable traits.[1]

The acknowledged expert on the subject of stress, Hans Selye, advised people to dwell on the pleasant aspects of life and on actions that can improve the situation.[2]

Confused, irrelevant, painful thoughts are invariably accompanied by stresses in the body and "knots" in the nervous system. We can sense them in our irregular breathing, in our distorted posture, in our strained body coordination, or our tortured facial expression. In other words, we no longer feel good in our body, and our Dan-Tien tells us to stop these useless, irrelevant, or harmful thoughts.

Conversely it is just as true that we think useful, relevant, and pleasant thoughts as soon as our breathing and our body coordination return to normal. As soon as we feel good in the body, our mind comes up with enjoyable thoughts that result in useful action.

When we live in tune with our Dan-Tien, we can forget about negative thoughts and negative psychology. We have no further need to dig into unhappy past experiences or into painful emotions. Instead we build on our successes and cultivate a harmonious state of mind/body. In this we are guided by the divine wisdom that we can sense in our center.

Pleasant Dreams

Suppose you have dreamed that a tree walks toward you, then turns into a dragon and swims across a river, where it is attacked by a motorcycle.

---

[1] Abraham Maslow, *Toward a Psychology of Being* (New York: Van Nos Reinhold, 1968).

[2] Hans Selye, *The Stress of Life* (New York: McGraw-Hill, 1956).

What does this tell you? Dreams mean something, no doubt. They reflect unconscious processes that the conscious mind has ignored or suppressed. They express something that you did not want to know during the day. This is why psychoanalysts ask their patients to tell their dreams. But when it comes to interpreting a particular dream, each analyst arrives at a different answer. Freudians see sex symbols in everything, and Jungians will look for archetypes. Some psychologists believe that only the dreamer can guess what the dream means.

In the context of Dan-Tien, you only need to ask one simple question: Was the dream pleasant or not? Did you wake up with a smile or a frown? Did your body feel relaxed and refreshed, or did you feel tense and confused?

If the dream involved any type of conflict or violence, or if you experienced any painful emotions, you can assume that you are at present ignoring or suppressing some sort of inner conflict. In the end it is you, the dreamer, who created the dream with its conflicts.

When you wake up and become aware of this, you may want to write down what happened in your dream. You can look upon it as a mysterious oracle, and you may or may not learn something from it. But the main lesson of a nasty dream is that you are somehow struggling against yourself. You can therefore treat the dream as you would any other negative thought or feeling: You can dissolve the underlying conflict by restoring the harmony in your Dan-Tien. Instead of analyzing or explaining it, you would go through the usual centering routine until you feel good again because the conflict has disappeared.

There is in fact not much difference between your waking and your dreaming thoughts. Even the thoughts you think right now are really "dreams," they are your subjective interpretations of reality.

By living in tune with your Dan-Tien, most of your dreams will be as pleasant as your days. At the same time your days will be more colorful because your conscious mind will be more creative. Just as in your dreams, you will transcend the limits of time and space in your daytime thinking. If your life is now a bit boring or one-dimensional, it can now become a "great dream."

The Dan-Tien Approach in a Nutshell

It is natural and normal to feel good and to enjoy every moment.

Digging into a problem and analyzing or explaining it while you feel tense and confused only creates more problems.

The first step must always be to find your center by gathering the Chi energy in your Dan-Tien. Once you feel good in your center, your mind will be able to explain everything—but not before.

When you notice unpleasant feelings in your Dan-Tien, you can ask yourself:

1) Are my energies centered, or are they nervously flitting around in my head and body?

2) Are my posture and movements centered, or are they awkward and strained? Are my belly muscles relaxed?

3) Do I enjoy every inbreath and outbreath, or is my breathing at the moment strained, shallow, short, or irregular?

4) Do I really enjoy what I am thinking and doing, or have negative emotions and useless, irrelevant thoughts crept in? Am I focused on what I am doing, or is my mind wandering about aimlessly?

If you answer "yes" to the first part of the above questions, you are on the right path. If, however, the answer is "yes" to the latter parts of these four questions, you have lost touch with the Dan-Tien. Once we are on the right track again we begin to see our past, our future, our relationships, and our projects in the right perspective, and we can take the course of action that "feels good" and gets results.

Feeling good in your center (Dan-Tien) means being on the right track (the Way of Tao). By being aware of your divine self, you feel good about yourself and your world. Everything you think and do makes sense and serves a purpose.

CHAPTER 14

Feeling Good is Good for You

Nature Wants Us to be Happy

We are endowed by Nature with an instinct that makes us seek pleasure and avoid pain. We increase our chances of survival by moving toward food, friendly company, love, and favorable environments, and by moving away from harmful influences. Joy and love have "survival value," as biologists have pointed out. To "feel good" is not a frivolous luxury as some scriptures suggest, but a biological need. When we follow the laws of Nature, she rewards us with joys and pleasures along the way.

Through millions of years of evolution humanity has developed this unconscious wisdom. Even our remote ancestors, the single-celled amoeba, had (and still has) this instinct to move toward food and favorable conditions, and to avoid hostile environments. These simple reflexes were then refined through the ages, especially in the higher animals. Human beings were furthermore endowed with an elaborate conscious mind that helps them to adapt to all kinds of conditions and to create their own environments through ingenious technology. The conscious mind enables us to think and reason, and it

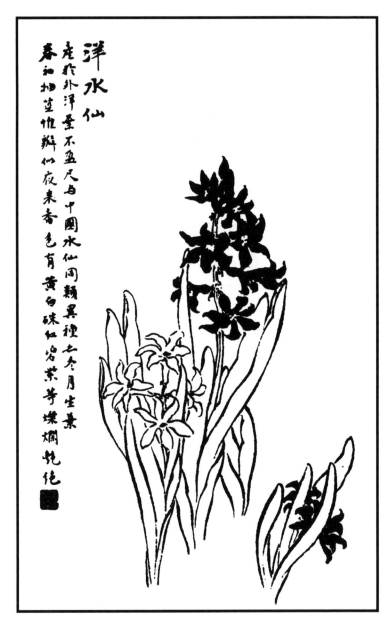

*Figure 21. We are endowed by Nature with
an instinct that makes us seek pleasure.*

distinguishes us from monkeys, dogs, or horses, for example. Although these higher animals can also think, they are not as adaptable and inventive as humans.

But the fact remains that our most vital functions take place on the unconscious level. Our survival depends on complex biological processes and on the animal wisdom that is contained in our nervous system, in our genes, and our cells. In many ways the body is more in touch with life than the conscious mind. While the mind can only grasp one thing at a time, the body can "sense" and process hundreds of things simultaneously. It has the sharp reflexes of a wild animal that is forever looking, feeling, searching, comparing, and choosing.

But most "civilized" people have been conditioned to ignore their instinctual wisdom and to live only by their intellect. They are no longer in touch with their unconscious power, and they have forgotten how to enjoy life. They violate the laws of Nature, and they are rewarded with suffering instead of joy. They need to rediscover their Dan-Tien to become fully human again.

Suffering is a Warning Signal

People who have lost touch with their Dan-Tien usually take their frustration, suffering, and unhappiness for granted. They feel that this is an unavoidable part of life, and they may quote sayings like:

> Good days are always followed by bad days.
> You have to take the bad with the good.
> We must struggle to get somewhere.
> Human beings are meant to suffer.
> It is noble to suffer and sacrifice for a good cause.
> Joy and sadness are two sides of a coin.
> It is immoral to enjoy life when others are suffering.
> We all have to bear our cross.

There is a grain of truth in such sayings of course. But suppose someone says: "Health and disease are two sides of a coin." This is also true in a way. Would we then assume that it is normal and natural to be sick half the time or to have a body that is half diseased? Would we believe that good health is always followed by disease, or that it is noble to be sick?

It is true that pain, suffering, and disease all have their function in life. They all come to us as teachers when we are on the wrong track. They first warn us, and when we don't listen they punish us. In this respect they are all beneficial and can lead to "enlightenment" for the person who has strayed from the path of physical or mental health. But to welcome pain, suffering, and disease because it is followed by health or happiness is like saying: "Please beat me and punish me because it feels so good when you stop." An element of sadomasochism is in fact part of this mentality.

But people who live in tune with their Dan-Tien use the pain/pleasure principle in the way intended by Nature. When they listen to their center for unpleasant sensations, they are really detecting pain in the beginning stages, before it starts to hurt. Then they use this subtle message to find their way back to normal, namely to the pleasant feeling of being at home in the body and in touch with the cosmic power Chi.

Happier Frames of Reference

In spite of what we may have been taught and what many experts say, we are not meant to struggle and suffer our way through life. But even after we have gained a basic understanding of the Dan-Tien concept, we may still have our doubts now and then. We may say, for example:

"To enjoy every minute or almost every minute is just impossible, because life has its ups and downs."

"The world in which we live today is so full of problems that we all get weighed down by them. All this suffering makes me sad."

"I have special problems with my lover/family/job/finances/ etc., that cannot be solved with such a recipe for instant happiness."

"My problems are deeply rooted in my past, and nothing can change my past. I will need years of thinking and/or counseling to get over them, and some problems will always remain."

"It is natural to be happy on some days and unhappy on others. This is what makes life exciting, and I wouldn't want it any other way."

"I think it is good to explode with anger, to shout and scream or to have a good cry, because this clears the air and makes me feel better."

"To grow and mature we need periods of suffering. All great minds had to struggle against overwhelming odds, and most creative people went through periods of madness."

All such arguments contain some truth. But they do not apply when we have been living in tune with our Dan-Tien for a while. When we practice the secret we soon notice that our life and our world have changed. There is a fundamental shift in emphasis. Some old beliefs that we used to take for granted fade away. New priorities emerge. Obsolete frames of reference are replaced by happier ones that are more in tune with life.

Past and future appear in a new light. Relationships become more meaningful and loving. We feel good about ourselves and our world, and we feel at home in the body. In time this becomes apparent in our posture, in the way we move and in our facial expression. We enjoy a higher degree of health and well-being, and we accomplish more with less effort.

Questions

But is it really wise to rely on these gut feelings all the time? Can body sensations be our main guide in life? Would it not be more noble to follow our conscience, to sacrifice ourselves for an ideal, and to make others happy first?

We do all this spontaneously when we are centered in the Dan-Tien. We are more aware of the needs of others, and we adhere to high standards. We are kind to others not because of some moral code or because we are afraid of punishment in hell, but because we enjoy helping others. We also enjoy contributing to a worthy cause.

But what about situations when we need self-discipline and endurance to attain a goal? When we are jogging or skiing, for instance, should we give up as soon as we feel some pain? When we have to do some unpleasant chore, should we just stop and relax whenever we feel strained? And when we want to lose weight, should we just give in to our physical urges and keep eating?

In the first example, when we are exerting ourselves physically, we can very well "feel good inside" while certain muscles ache. But if our sporting activities do not feel good inside, we may ask ourselves if they are really recreation or whether we are indulging in a form of self-punishment. We can easily improve our fitness without much strain, over-exertion, or self-discipline, if we choose an activity we enjoy. We can build up our strength gradually without pushing ourselves. Some people stay fit just by dancing, walking, and swimming now and then.

As for the second example, there will be times when we have to exert ourselves to finish an unpleasant task. But if this creates unhappy feelings, we may ask ourselves if it is the task that makes us unhappy or our attitude toward it. Do we perhaps feel that we chose the wrong career? Do we resent our colleagues, do we hate the boss? Or did we forget to rest now and then or get out of a tense posture? These are the kinds of problems that we can detect and clear up by listening to our Dan-Tien.

In the third example, when we want to lose weight, the overeating definitely makes us feel bad in the Dan-Tien, although it may tickle our taste buds. It is our habit of ignoring the Dan-Tien that makes us eat too much. Self-discipline is not the answer as long as we are not aware of the body's needs. When we live in tune with the Dan-Tien, we know what is good for the body. We are no longer tempted to gorge ourselves with junk food to make up for our feelings of inner emptiness, lack of love, resentment, loneliness, envy, or whatever. We are free to satisfy our hunger for life in more natural and enjoyable ways. The same goes for all other addictions, from smoking, workaholism, and alcoholism to dependence on legal or illegal drugs.

Facing the Issues

Another question: Shouldn't we face unpleasant issues squarely, even if it hurts? Aren't we evading problems and conflicts when we follow the Dan-Tien and try to enjoy every minute? Aren't we taking the easy way out by looking only at the sunny side of life?

Quite the contrary: Only when we feel good inside can we be certain that we are facing the right issues in the right way. When we enjoy what we are thinking or doing we know for sure that we are not wasting our time and that we are making good use of the opportunities that life offers at the moment.

As long as we feel friction in the Dan-Tien, we can assume that our picture of reality is distorted, that we are using the wrong concepts, that our timing is wrong, or that we are somehow on the wrong track.

These are the things that we have not been taught at school or elsewhere. Boys and girls in our culture are not really supposed to feel good. Instead they are constantly reminded that they must control themselves, that they must please the teachers and parents first of all, and that they must struggle their way through school. They must be obedient and memorize whatever they are told in order to get good grades, under threat of punishment. By the time they leave school, most of them have lost their natural curiosity, creativity, and spontaneity.

People who have been programmed to ignore their feelings do not get good grades in the school of life. To pass the tests of real life they have to unlearn many of the things that they learned in school and other coercive institutions, and they have to rediscover their Dan-Tien.

Perverse Pleasures

But what about people who find perverse pleasure in stealing, torturing, or killing? What about sadists, masochists, rapists, and sex perverts? Is it not true that Nature misguides them by rewarding them with joy for their strange pursuits? Are they not living proof of the fact that our gut feelings often lead us astray? How can we put our faith in the Dan-Tien concept when our instinct for doing what feels good can go so terribly wrong?

Actually it is the other way around: All these people have lost touch with their center; they are victims of repressed negative emotions. Deep down they are confused, frustrated, and unhappy, although they may not admit it. Their pleasures are very mixed indeed, they are only poor substitutes for real happiness, they are miserable attempts to escape from a life of unhappiness now and then. This goes for the majority of such people, although there may be rare cases of incurable insanity. Most of them would gladly give up their "pleasures" if they knew how to attain the real pleasures that come naturally to anyone who knows the secret of Dan-Tien.

In fact we have to admit that there is a "pervert" in all of us, because we all lose touch with our center now and then. We are all dominated by "sick" thoughts or emotions from time to time. In these moments we are punished by Nature, we suffer and we harm ourselves and those around us.

Perversion cannot really be eradicated by laws and the threat of torture, prison, death, or punishment in hell. People change only when they are offered rewards that are more tempting than the ones presently enjoyed. Misguided and confused people can only give up their perverse pleasures if they are convinced that they can easily attain much greater pleasures.

But nobody ever showed them how to enjoy life the natural way. Since childhood they have been told that good children, good students, and good citizens must ignore their feelings and endure the inner pain, that they must not think or talk about the body below the belt. Now they are hooked on negative habits and alienated from their bodies, and they look for pleasure in the wrong places.

Instead of blaming them we could try to teach them the secret of Dan-Tien. They might really get a kick out of that and get addicted to the pleasure of enjoying every minute.

Familiar Phrases

We can detect negative states by being aware of our Dan-Tien. We can also "hear" them by listening to the way we talk. When we talk to ourselves or to others, we often use familiar phrases like "that's really something" or "here we go again" or "that's the way it goes."

Some of these are harmless little additions to our speech, but in others we can detect a negative note. Some of them really "do not feel good." We can notice this when others use them. For instance, if George says, "I am doing everything wrong again," we know that he has slipped into the negative state. We may also sense this from the defeated tone of his voice, his facial expression, his breathing, the position of his neck and head, his posture, or his gestures. When Joan says, "I just hate this man," we can also assume that she is in a negative state just now.

It is usually futile to point this out to people who are not familiar with the Dan-Tien concept. To them, such habitual phrases seem natural and logical, they express how they feel about things "as they really are." Through their negative frame of mind they are inviting problems, conflicts, failure, or even accidents. When the inevitable then happens, they will say, "You see, I told you that these things always happen to me!"

But what about yourself? Do you sometimes use negative phrases, to others or yourself, such as, "I'm not good at this," "I could kill you," "Nobody understands me," "I just hate this," "This always happens to me," "I'll shoot myself," "People are stupid"?

Sentences that contain nasty four-letter words usually reveal negative states. They originate in an unhappy mind and are meant to accuse or embarrass.

People who are not familiar with the Dan-Tien practice may insist that all such phrases are just harmless ways of letting off steam. Nasty toilet expressions, for instance, tend to be popular with people who went through severe toilet training in early childhood. Nasty sex expressions are more often used by people who grew up in prudish societies. Nasty blasphemies are more common among people who feel inhibited by negative religion or false morality.

All such phrases are therefore justified in some way. But people do not really feel good in their Dan-Tien when they use them. They may claim that they are having fun, but deep down they know that they are unhappy about themselves, about others, and about life in general.

Beliefs that Feel Good

All of the major religions contain much wisdom. All of them also harbor certain traps that can hinder us in our pursuit of happiness and success. We must keep in mind that our traditional beliefs evolved along lines that suited the prevailing political systems and power structures. Quite often the official religions were bent and twisted to conform to the interests of certain rulers, despots, land owners, ruling classes, or majorities with their vested interests. Other beliefs that did not fit in were suppressed or eliminated in the course of centuries.

The Catholic Church, for example, tortured millions of women to death and confiscated their property during the Middle Ages. These women did not conform to the male-oriented teachings of Rome. The Hindu religion considers the caste system "sacred" because it preserves the privileges of the upper castes. Muslims proudly claim to have a classless society, but they treat women as second-class citizens. Most Buddhist sects believe in political tolerance, but they admonish their followers to do their duty, to obey the ruler, to endure the sadness and suffering of life in silence, and not to expect too much from this life.

Many religious mythologies were created or promoted to explain and justify the beliefs that suited certain rulers. Gods were modeled after kings, local chiefs, or despots. Opposing gods or goddesses were declared satanic, and their followers were persecuted or killed. In the male-oriented monotheistic religions of the West we find myths that "prove" that the world was created by a male god and that women are inadequate and immoral. Hinduism contains many myths that "prove" the inferiority of the Untouchable Caste, by claiming that these people have committed crimes in previous lives. Buddhist texts "prove" that suffering and unhappiness must be accepted as normal and natural. A Jewish prayer for men lets them say: "Thank you, oh God, for making me a man and not a woman." Muslim scriptures "prove" that every man has the right and the duty to beat his wife if he thinks that she has strayed from the path of the Koran.

Similar, but more subtle, beliefs can be found in most authoritarian organizations, in military units, school systems, businesses, and also in families. They are usually interwoven with wise quotations and eternal truths that nobody can dispute or doubt. In this way the impression is created that the myth must also be true.

How can we separate the wisdom from the lies, the wheat from the chaff? If we were to analyze all relevant beliefs intellectually, this would take a lifetime. But fortunately there is a simpler way: Our Dan-Tien can tell us whether a belief is in tune with life or not. When a belief or custom disagrees with our natural and spontaneous impulses and keeps making us feel bad instead of good, we can regard this as a warning signal. By living in tune with our center, we can gradually eliminate the unnatural elements of any belief. When we feel good about our beliefs again we are on the right track. This good feeling will be reflected in everything we think and do, right here and now.

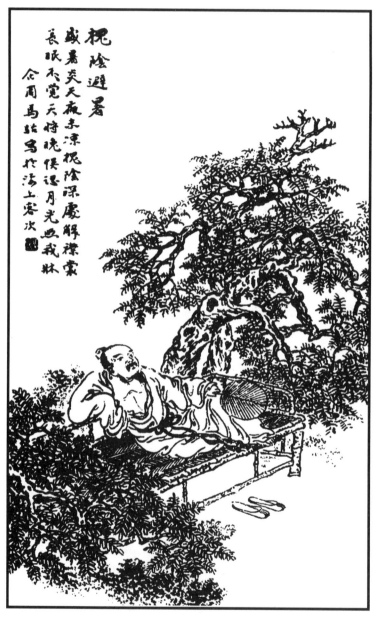

Figure 22. We can get into the habit of enjoying (almost) every minute of each day.

CHAPTER 15

At Home in the Body

Body Harmony

Thoughts that do not feel good are not worth pursuing. Unpleasant sensations in the Dan-Tien invariably tell us that we are on the wrong track somehow. The same applies to our everyday activities. When we do not feel good while walking, sitting, standing, or breathing, we can assume that we are doing these things in the wrong way. The body then does not function optimally and gracefully, but strains and struggles because of inner friction.

We may be tempted to think that it does not really matter whether we enjoy these "basic body functions." After all, we walk to get from A to B, we sit down to get the weight off our feet and we breathe to get oxygen into our system. Why should we expect to get much pleasure out of these things?

In the same way we may do gymnastics, jogging, aerobics, or Yoga to stay fit and healthy, even if we find it unpleasant or painful. We may endure beauty treatments or life-extending cures, or spend great sums of money to rejuvenate ourselves in health resorts. Then we go home and live as before, straining and doing things in ways that we do not really enjoy.

To get out of this dismal cycle is easy if we follow the subtle messages from our Dan-Tien. Gradually we can learn to adopt pleasant ways of walking, sitting, standing, and breathing, simply by sensing our way until it feels good. Just as we can drop unpleasant thoughts or emotions, we can also drop unpleasant postures and breathing habits. Without much need for special programs or exercises we can get into the habit of enjoying (almost) every minute of each day.

By doing this we are also exercising the body without formal exercises. Simply by letting the body function in a natural and enjoyable way for 16 hours each day, we keep it quite fit and healthy. This adds to our good looks and extends our life expectancy automatically. Our need for medicines, doctors, health resorts, and health insurance is drastically reduced or even eliminated.

Moving Naturally

People who live close to nature can usually be recognized by their graceful, animal-like movements, and their dignified posture. There is a spring in their step, their spines are straight but flexible, and their head balances on top of the spine. Just by looking at them we can sense that they feel happy and at home in the body.

Sometimes, when we walked in nature, we have also experienced such a pleasant state. But next day, when we returned to our everyday routine at home and at work, the harmony was soon lost again.

It seems that somehow we are always rushing about, trying to be somewhere else, pushing ourselves. Even when we have enough time, we worry about the future and tense our body in anticipation. We tend to stretch the head forward impatiently and forget to breathe properly.

This stress in the body distorts the mind also, it creates useless thoughts. We tell ourselves, for instance, that we must do things that are really irrelevant or harmful. We think we must get there and do this and that before we can afford the luxury of relaxing and feeling good. We think that we must force the body to reach some far-fetched goal. As soon as we reach that goal we rush on toward the next one, and so on. We think that such goals justify our habit of straining and suffering.

This mentality, which is more prevalent in the West than in the East, makes peace of mind and the enjoyment of graceful body movements almost impossible. In the long run it distorts the posture permanently, and puts destructive stress on joints and ligaments, especially around the spine. Here lies the main reason for the catastrophic increase of joint and spine problems in our society.

This is why some people in show business and politics, who must present a favorable image, attend special schools where they learn to move, walk, stand, and sit naturally and gracefully. The Alexander Method, for instance, teaches them how to let the head "float" on top of the spine, instead of stretching it forward. Then they learn how to relax head, neck, throat, and shoulders, and how to breathe from the diaphragm at the bottom of the lungs. Slowly they drop the habit of straining and regain confidence in the body. The result is a more dynamic, graceful, and dignified appearance. Other ways of accomplishing this include the age-old Chinese technique of Tai Chi Chuan that keeps people fit through slow, dance-like movements.

Posture Checklist

Whenever your posture "does not feel good," experiment until the unpleasant sensation disappears. Here is a list of critical points:

- Tilt your hips into "horizontal" position until stomach muscles relax. The ring formed by your belt should be horizontal, not tilting forward or backward.
- If an imaginary bowl were placed on the ring of your belt and filled with water, the water should not spill in any direction while you stand or walk.
- Imagine a thread pulling you up from the top of your head, so that your spine is straightened, and you get a feeling of floating as you walk.

✿ Let your arms drop at the shoulders and relax your neck. Let arms swing freely as you walk.

✿ Now and then turn your palms forward and outward, which causes your upper spine to straighten and your lungs to open.

✿ Balance your head on top of the spine, avoid stretching it forward. Keep your eyes relaxed and mobile, avoid staring.

✿ Accentuate exhaling all the way, then let the breath come spontaneously. Your lungs are empty when you can no longer talk.

✿ Do some bending and stretching occasionally, to keep the body young and the spine flexible. Find some enjoyable activity that requires you to bend and stretch to the limit, such as gardening, dancing, swimming, or aerobics.

✿ When you feel a pleasant tingle along your spine, you know that you have found the right dynamic balance.

✿ Enjoy every moment and every movement.

Sitting Comfortably

Most people nowadays spend at least half of their time sitting—while eating, working, traveling, driving, reading, talking, or watching television. Even if we move around more than the average person, we will spend hours each day in a sitting position. Therefore we may as well ensure that sitting for us is a pleasure and not a necessary evil.

Sitting need not cause aches, shallow breathing, a sagging figure, and feelings of fatigue, reduced well-being, or discomfort. Such things happen only when we ignore the subtle signals from our body. By living in tune with the Dan-Tien we can avoid bad sitting habits, just as we can avoid painful emotions or useless thoughts. The goal is always the same—to avoid unpleasant or unnatural states of mind and body. The answer is always to keep exploring and shifting until we feel good again.

We can adopt "active" sitting habits, as opposed to rigid or slumping positions. We can rediscover the instinct that tells us what the body needs at any given time. We can follow the urge to stretch or get up and walk around as often as possible or convenient. If we are on our own we can even sing and dance now and then, whenever we feel that mind and body begin to stagnate. We may even ask ourselves if we have to sit at all. Quite often we can do the job standing or lying down!

We can learn from small children. They still have straight spines, they enjoy sitting or squatting on the floor, and they seldom stay in the same position for long. They do not yet have back problems that most of us develop later in life. Spinal problems are seldom inherited, they are the result of bad posture and a lack of exercise.

If we want to meditate or practice Zen, there is no need to torture ourselves with pretzel postures. While people who grow up in the Orient find the squatting position natural and comfortable, Westerners can reach the state of inner union also while sitting normally. One solution is described in chapter 6—sitting on two firm pillows and using a third one to lean against a wall.

Checklist for Sitting

❦ Develop "active" sitting habits, avoid stagnation. Do not just endure uncomfortable postures, but shift now and then until you feel good again.

❦ Try to find a chair that feels comfortable for longer periods. Use firm pillows to put your body in the right position if necessary.

❦ Keep neck and eyes relaxed. A frozen neck and staring eyes are a sure sign of mental tension and confusion.

❦ When sitting at a table to eat or work, keep your spine fairly vertical. Let your head balance on top of the spine, avoid leaning over your work or food whenever possible.

❦ In everything you do, remember that your gravity center lies in your pelvis, not in your head or your chest. Just being aware of this will balance your posture.

❦ You are doing it right when you find that you enjoy every moment.

Why do so many people have bent spines? At birth they had normal backbones, and the curve developed later in life. But why would they adopt a posture that is neither enjoyable, nor efficient, nor good-looking? Were they perhaps afraid of relaxing and enjoying life, or did they feel that straining and struggling is virtuous?

To drop this habit and let the spine straighten out may take a long time, and spinal exercises may help. But what is needed most of all is the conviction that good posture feels good in the Dan-Tien because it is natural and normal.

Breathing is a Pleasure

When we think and act in tune with life, we experience our breathing as joyful. Whenever we notice that our breathing is no longer pleasant and refreshing, we have lost some of our inner harmony. And when we experience our breathing as tense or unpleasant, we can be sure that we are on the wrong track somehow, that we are harboring painful emotions and that we are thinking useless or harmful thoughts.

By following the signals of our Dan-Tien we can find our way back into a natural breathing rhythm. We can feel our way until each breath feels good again. When we are active outdoors, for example, our breathing tends to normalize quite soon. Especially when we walk in beautiful natural surroundings, we breathe deeply and rhythmically, and the feeling of well-being returns. But chances are that we spend much of our time indoors or in man-made surroundings. How can we maintain pleasant breathing habits under the conditions of modern life?

The first thing to remember is that we can only feel good when each breath originates from the bottom of our lungs near the body's gravity center in the belly. Nervous people breathe from the middle of the chest. People who have lost touch with life and with the Dan-Tien breathe in short gasps from the shoulders, with tense neck and face muscles. By breathing from our center we have access to an inexhaustible source of Chi life energy.

The temptation to breathe superficially is greatest when we pay close attention to something, when we concentrate on a task, or when we are stuck with some tense thought. But as soon as the tension is resolved, we breathe a sigh of relief or, if we have felt somewhat upset, we exhale convulsively in the form of laughter. This is why laughing, singing, or humming gets us back into a pleasant breathing rhythm.

How often do you exhale in one minute while you are resting? With most adults the breathing rate per minute (BPM) fluctuates around 15–20. The larger the lungs, the slower should be the breath. After you have adopted the Dan-Tien habit for some months, your rate will probably drop to 10 or even lower.

Breathing Checklist

Tense and irregular breathing is always accompanied by painful emotions and useless thoughts. By being in touch with your Dan-Tien, you develop pleasant habits of thinking, feeling, and breathing, and you laugh more often.

- ☗ Laughter feels good because it empties the lungs and gets you back into a natural breathing rhythm.
- ☗ Singing, humming, dancing, or hopping around can also get you back into the habit of exhaling all the way.
- ☗ Accentuate the outbreath instead of taking deep breaths. After the lungs are really empty, the inbreath follows spontaneously and joyfully.
- ☗ Abdominal breathing, from the belly and not from the chest, feels good and also stimulates your digestion. Mental and physical stagnation and constipation is often the result of shallow breathing.
- ☗ Rest and sleep can also help to normalize your breathing, especially after tense and hectic periods.
- ☗ You are doing it right when you find that you are enjoying each breath.

Sleeping Well

We spend one third of our life asleep in bed, and our general well-being depends to a great extent on how well we sleep. Restless nights, sleeplessness, nightmares, and hangovers in the morning can take much of the fun out of life.

A good night's sleep is necessary to rejuvenate the mind/body and to prepare it for the challenges of the day. By using a little common sense we can make sure that we wake up feeling good and ready to go each morning.

Sleeping Checklist

◆ Get into a relaxed state of mind/body before falling asleep. Stretch out your limbs and relax all muscles. Think pleasant thoughts and relax your eyes. Try "exhaling through the soles of your feet" as described in chapter 6.

◆ Find a sleeping position that lets you feel good in your Dan-Tien and at home in your body. You will be surprised to find that even in bed your posture can make all the difference in the way you feel.

◆ Eat little or nothing the three hours before going to sleep. Supper should be light and easily digested. Many a bad dream or nightmare, or hangover is caused by a heavy evening meal.

◆ Drinking any liquid with your supper can cause fermentation and gases. This may disturb your sleep and make you feel groggy in the morning.

◆ You will breathe more easily during sleep if you limit the use of stimulants, irritants, spices, and drugs. Especially alcohol and nicotine tend to narrow your breathing channels and cause an anxious feeling during the night.

◆ Most people sleep better when they avoid lying on the left side, since this can impede the blood flow from the heart.

◆ With overweight people the big stomach pushes up against their lungs as soon as they lie down, which interferes with breathing. This is one more reason for staying slim and eating light in the evening. Heavy food eaten just before going to sleep is converted mostly into fat, not energy.

❧ When you sleep well and wake up refreshed next morning, you feel great and have no need for stimulants like caffeine or nicotine to pep you up. Life itself offers plenty of excitement.

Eating and Excreting

With each breath we take in oxygen, and we also expel carbon dioxide and other waste products. In ecological terms, this benefits not only us but also the plant life around us. All plants and trees need the carbon dioxide exhaled by humans and animals, and in turn they produce the oxygen we need.

This process of absorbing and expelling is vital. Our life literally depends on it, and this is why Nature rewards correct breathing with joy. Another aspect of this is the taking in of nutrients (eating), the assimilation of food (digesting), and the excretion of waste products (going to the toilet).

Eating and drinking is pleasant, of course. But what about the digesting and excreting? Even here, Nature has seen to it that these important functions are experienced as pleasant, although to a lesser extent. Only people who are sick or who eat the wrong foods find digestion and excretion unpleasant or painful.

If the body does not regularly eliminate waste products through the lungs by exhaling, through the skin by perspiring, and through the stool and urine in the toilet, we soon begin to feel uncomfortable. When these toxic wastes accumulate over longer periods, they literally poison us. Most chronic diseases and most diseases of civilization are partly or wholly due to self-intoxication by the body's own waste products. The bacteria that thrive on these wastes are then mistakenly blamed as the cause of a disease. An overfed and under-exercised body is invariably full of poisons, and this is why some people are healthier in hard times than in times of ease and affluence.

Until recently the subject of excretion was taboo, and people were even ashamed to admit that they went to the toilet at all.

But nowadays we can accept all our bodily functions as normal, desirable, and enjoyable.

Much of our time every day is spent buying or producing food, preparing it and eating it. This becomes especially obvious during periods of fasting, when we find that we have "nothing much to do" much of the time, and that we have many extra hours at our disposal. On such occasions we realize how much our life revolves around our physical needs and pleasures, and how little we cultivate the more subtle joys that life offers.

Dancing is Fun

Since time began men and women have enjoyed dancing to beautiful music. Dancing also happens to be the ideal way to keep fit. While most other exercises make us feel tired or bored even before we begin, dancing is fun. Normally we would dance with a partner. But if there is nobody around, it is fun to dance alone, too. Children do it all the time, in a sheer expression of joy and vitality.

But do we really need all that exercise? The experts agree that we need to keep active. The body was not designed for a sedentary or stationary way of life. If we do not exercise at least fifteen minutes about once a day, fat collects in the tissues, veins, and around the heart and other organs. Our blood circulation gets sluggish, our breathing gets shallow, our whole metabolism begins to stagnate—and our mind gets nervous and inefficient in the process. Needless to say, all this does not improve our looks either. What we call "good looks" is largely a matter of healthy skin, hair and teeth, of posture and fitness in general.

An occasional swim, a long walk or visits to the health club may be a good idea. But what the body really needs is daily vigorous stimulation. This we can get the easy way by dancing at home or elsewhere, alone or with others. The right rhythm and joyous atmosphere is best created through bouncy music. Just hopping around in a kind of double step does it: right–left, left–right, right–left, left–right. The movements flow easily from the gravity center, from the Dan-Tien.

On the first day we may be out of breath after a few minutes. But gradually our condition improves, and after one month we wonder how we could have been so weak in the beginning. There is no need to force the body. But people with heart conditions or other ailments should consult their doctor first.

To vary the routine we can invent our own dances and add some stretching movements here and there. We can swing our arms and legs in various ways, twist the spine and neck to the rhythm. The body will tell us where we need to strengthen our weak points. We can hum, sing, or even yodel if we feel like it. If we start today, we will notice the difference in a few days, and soon we regain the fitness and vitality we had as children.

Dan-Tien—Better than Drugs

There are only two reasons why people take drugs—to make them feel good or to kill pain. People take drugs for "kicks" when they feel bored, for peace of mind when they feel frustrated, for relaxation when they feel tense, and for happiness when they feel unhappy. This is true of all legal and illegal drugs, including alcohol, Prozac, marijuana, hashish, LSD, opium, cocaine, and heroin. The effect does not last, of course, and ever stronger doses are needed to stay "high."

The need for drugs arises because in our society we are not taught how to feel good without such chemical crutches to maintain a state of inner harmony. With our outer-oriented mentality we are forever trying to master the environment and to manipulate the mind/body. We are helpless victims of painful emotions and harmful thought patterns. In our desperation we turn to mind-altering chemicals that promise to make us feel good again.

Drugs promise to help "uptight" people to relax and find themselves, to discard false identities, to overcome inhibitions. They promise lonely people to get over the feeling of alienation. They promise uprooted people to find their roots.

Most drugs are taken to reduce tension and to cope with the stresses of everyday life. High-pressure salesmen crave a strong drink to unwind after work. Intellectuals take LSD to break out of their artificial mental structures. Middle class youngsters smoke pot to shake off their phony suburban identity and their parents' preoccupation with superficial values.

More and more people believe that there is a chemical for every problem. In the USA alone, three tons of aspirin are taken every day, and every year 120 million prescriptions for psycho-active drugs are filled; 30 million Americans take tranquilizers, and 20 million take stimulants. Americans spend over 140 billion dollars ($140,000,000,000) on illegal drugs each year. This includes 180 tons of cocaine, 12 tons of heroin, and over 30,000 tons of marijuana. Even more serious are the consequences of legal drug abuse: 400,000 Americans die from the effects of smoking every year, and 100,000 from the effects of drinking.

Most addicts feel that drugs are the only way to solve individual or social problems, to handle the pressures of modern life and to "be themselves." But drugs can only replace one artificiality with another, and they interfere with the self-balancing forces of the mind/body. They can be beneficial only in the hands of those who can take them or leave them. But such people prefer not to bother with them because they have access to the "real thing," the inner harmony they attain by living in tune with the Dan-Tien.

The more artificial and violent a society becomes, the more alcoholics and drug addicts it will tend to produce. Addiction is seldom the cause of mental and social ills, but a symptom and a warning signal. It tells us that our culture, our concept of the world, and our way of life have lost touch with the central source of life. Here is a list of other symptoms:

We overemphasize the intellect at the expense of subtle intuition. We are preoccupied with external reality and superficial values, and neglect our inner creative potential. We tend to think in terms of either-or, of struggle and conflict, and we are unable to resolve dichotomies and problems. We prefer male (Yang) values, violent sports, violent entertainment and male deities, at the expense of female (Yin) values, enjoyment of nature, and appreciation of "Mother Earth." Our attitude toward the body is hostile and our medicine is mechanistic. We do not utilize inner healing powers. We neglect our need for deep love and affection, and view sex as a sport or a diversion, or as a salable commodity. We prefer artificial social structures that are controlled from above according to the patriarchal model, instead of letting organic and democratic structures crystallize from within.

In short, we find here all the signs of a society that makes it difficult for the individual to live in tune with the Dan-Tien.

Mental and Dental Health

By living in tune with the Dan-Tien we get into the habit of enjoying every minute. Just as we can learn to ride a bicycle, to swim, or to brush our teeth, so we can learn to keep our mind/body fit and uncluttered and largely free of painful emotions.

The parallels between brushing teeth and clearing the mind are in fact remarkable. Some twenty years ago an American dentist[1] developed a method for completely eliminating tooth decay and gum disease. All his patients, which numbered twenty thousand at the time, were freed from dental problems for the rest of their lives, except for the twice-yearly removal of plaque and tartar. I adopted the method myself and wrote a book about it ten years ago, and I have had no dental problems since.[2]

Did the fraternity of dentists congratulate him on this remarkable achievement and learn from his approach? Far from it. They were afraid of losing their lucrative incomes, and they tried to put him out of business. He was sued by the American Dental Association for "practicing an unrecognized specialty," namely prevention. Fortunately this resulted in a great deal of publicity, and he was invited to appear on dozens of radio and television shows. He also wrote hundreds of articles and several books on the subject.

---

[1] Robert O. Nara, *Dental Self-Sufficiency* (Lake Linder, MI: Oramedics, 1975). If you want to write for a copy, write to R.R.1, Box 112, Lake Linder, MI, 49945.

[2] Christopher Markert, *So Pflege ich meine Zähne* (Munich, Germany: Goldman Verlag, 1983).

When I interviewed dentists in several countries while doing research for my book, I encountered the same resentment and professional jealousy. Many dentists got angry when they heard about the method, and none of them wanted to know how it worked. They merely wanted to continue their practice as usual, although they knew that their patients would lose one tooth after another, until they needed expensive dentures.

Such vested interests are also at work in the field of psychology, and the book you are reading now will be condemned by most psychologists, because it teaches people to enjoy life without their help. Self-sufficiency and self-reliance are bad for business, and they undermine the prestige of the "experts." Psychologists, as well as dentists and other doctors, like to believe that their methods are infallible and irreplaceable, even if they treat only the symptoms, and even if the patient does not really benefit in the end.

CHAPTER 16

The Happy Child Within

Rediscovering the Child Within

When we live in tune with the Dan-Tien we naturally harmonize with young children because we are in touch with the inner child. To rediscover the inner child we do not have to analyze and explain our childhood. What matters is not so much our past but our present attitude toward it.

How do we feel about childhood and children in general? If we are in the habit of rejecting our own childhood, we may have mixed feelings about children also. Perhaps we have been influenced by certain theories and practices that prevail in our culture. Perhaps we assume that our customary ways of handling babies and of raising and educating children are quite all right.

But as we begin to live more in tune with our Dan-Tien in all areas of life, we may begin to doubt certain things that we are now taking for granted. Here and there we may stumble over ideas and practices that do not "feel good." Gradually we may want to replace these with others that are more in tune

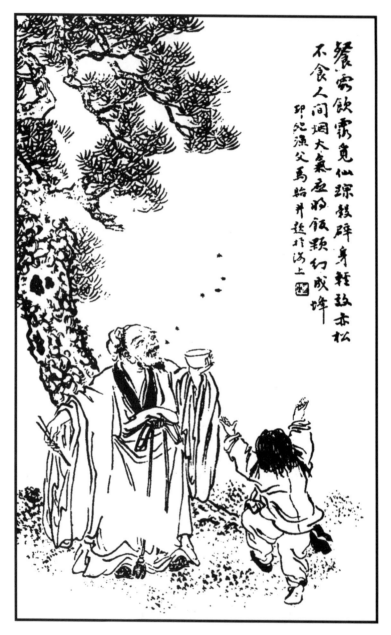

Figure 23. We naturally harmonize with young children.

with human nature. This will then enable us to appreciate children in general and the child within us in particular.

Children in the Far East

People in the Far East see children in a different light. Their lives revolve around the family, not around the individual and his/her achievements. Children are the essence of the family, not an addition to it. The contemporary Chinese/American, Lin Yutang, compared Western and Far-Eastern societies and came to this conclusion: "It has seemed to me that the final test of any civilization is, what type of husbands and wives and fathers and mothers does it turn out? Besides the austere simplicity of such a question, every other achievement of civilization—art, philosophy, literature, and material living—pales to insignificance."[1]

The famous I Ching, the "Bible" of the Far East, is really about a family consisting of father, mother, three sons and three daughters, and their relationships with each other. In the Western Bible we find a universe that is created by an unmarried father whose son is also unmarried. Parts of our Bible help us to understand and appreciate children. Others do the opposite, and some of them make us wince. We can sense that they originated with people who condemned children because they hated themselves. Whereas Jesus enjoyed the company of children and admonished his followers to become like children if they wanted to enter the Kingdom of Heaven, Western culture as a whole reflects a quite different attitude. St. Paul taught that children come into the world as sinners because they are the result of the sinful sex act. To this day, many people in the West feel that children are little savages and sinners who must be guided through strict discipline, a spiritual life, and the threat of punishment until they become real Christians.

---

[1] Lin Yutang, *The Importance of Living* (London: Wm. Heinemann, 1938), p. 149.

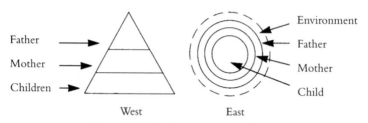

Figure 24. The family East and West.

In the Far East, the family resembles a circle with the child in the center, whereas the Western family looks more like a pyramid with the children at the bottom (see figure 24).

Happy Children

The Far-Eastern attitude toward children is also shared by most Indian tribes in North and South America, whose remote ancestors had migrated from Asia. When American Indians first met white settlers, they were often appalled at the callous and cruel ways in which the whites treated their own children.

Some years ago an American anthropologist[2] made similar observations with the Indians of Venezuela. In remote jungles she came upon tribes that had never seen white people before. The Indians led a simple life, of the type that we associate with the Stone Age. But what impressed the anthropologist was their inexplicable happiness. What was their secret? Were they using a hitherto unknown drug? Was their religion in any way special? Had they developed an unusually harmonious social structure?

These people seemed to enjoy everything they did, even the most strenuous tasks, and they hardly ever argued with each other. When work had to be done, nobody seemed to be in charge, but somehow the work got done spontaneously. While the members of the expedition worried, argued, cursed, and suffered often, the Indians kept displaying this "irrational" happiness.

They seemed to be free of the "everyday frustration" and neurotic symptoms that we consider normal in Western societies.

---

[2] Jean Liedloff, *The Continuum Concept* (New York: Warner Books, 1977).

With growing amazement Liedloff, the anthropologist, watched them day after day, week after week, trying to discover the reason for the "abnormal" behavior. As she was taking notes one day, she suddenly noticed something about the Indian babies.[3] They were not the hyperactive brats, the screaming, annoying bundles of frustration that she remembered from her native New York. What she saw instead were serene, smiling little people.

Why were they smiling? Apparently they were treated in a special way by their mothers and other members of the family and tribe. Most of the time during the day they were carried on their mother's back while she went about her daily tasks. When the baby got restless, it was swung around and breast-fed. At night it slept next to the mother and father in the same bed. Thus it grew up in an atmosphere of continuous love and contact.

At the moment of birth, this baby had not been exposed to harsh lights, loud voices, and chemical disinfectants. It had not been manhandled and slapped by a (male) gynecologist to make it scream. After birth it had not been isolated in a separate room or plastic box, left alone to endure the terror of loneliness. Later it was not kept in a crib or baby carriage for endless hours. When it screamed and squirmed from pain, hunger, or loneliness, it was never purposely left alone to let it develop its voice or to let it get used to the hard facts of life.

Therefore it felt deep down that it could trust others, that it was loved and appreciated by those around it. The world was a good place to be born into, and it was good to be alive. A baby like this will spontaneously try to please others, it will soon develop into a happy member of the family and the tribe.

When it grows up it will not feel an irrational craving for recognition and ego-satisfaction that is so common with people in Western societies who have suffered from maternal deprivation. It will not be compelled by an obsessive, all-consuming desire to amass huge fortunes, to collect more and more academic titles or military medals, or to acquire more and more fame and power merely to satisfy the craving for love and recognition that

---

[3] Liedloff, p. 18.

it lacked as a baby. Instead it will grow up to become a happy, sane, and responsible adult, and a loving mother or father.

People who grow up in this way will know instinctively and spontaneously how to bring up their own children. Unlike parents in the "civilized" countries who have lost this self-reliance, they will need no books or expert advice on how to raise happy children.

Liedloff mentions in passing that the tribe she studied had a "matrilineal" social structure, as opposed to the patriarchal Western society from which she came.[4] She observed that, when a young Indian couple decided to live together, the man usually moved in with the woman's family. Similar customs are also found with most North and South American Indians and in Tibet. Family life in these tribes tends to center around the mother, and the children usually feel more attached to the maternal clan. The father's role is also important, but he spends most of his time outside in the jungle, hunting, fishing, and exploring.

Such tribes do not need a fixed social order imposed from above by a strong authoritarian leader, and they do not normally believe in an almighty male god. Instead, the people live together in a more or less spontaneous and organic family arrangement based on blood ties, mutual affection, and convenience.

Liedloff noticed one exception in this idyllic world. One man often wandered around with a frown on his face and did not enjoy most of the communal activities. It turned out that he had been raised in a missionary school in the nearest town. There he had to follow strict rules and a rigid work schedule. Consequently he had lost his initiative and developed an aversion against work. Now the tribe felt sorry for him, but everybody hoped that he would soon rediscover the joy of working with others.[5]

Birth Without Violence

In the West it is taken for granted that birth is a traumatic experience. Babies are born screaming, with faces contorted from the

---

[4] Liedloff, p. 22.
[5] Liedloff, p. 22, 112

terror of being pushed out of the safe womb into the world of harsh realities. Psychologists such as Arthur Janov have even built an entire theory around the birth experience. He lets his patients relive their birth and re-enact their "primal scream." This, he says, helps them to get rid of repressed anguish and other accumulated pain, and to free themselves of hangups and neuroses. This is a variation of the Freudian approach and it has the same limitations, as mentioned in chapter 13.

But the trauma of birth need not be cured at all—if it can be prevented in the first place. This is what a French doctor found. In his travels through certain parts of India, Dr. Frederick Leboyer observed how babies were born happy, smiling, sometimes actually laughing within hours. In his classic book *Birth Without Violence*,[6] he describes and illustrates with photos how these babies are delivered gently, in subdued light. They are then immediately placed on the mother's belly, where they feel warm and secure. Later they are placed in a bath of lukewarm water.

For months before birth, the mother has prepared herself through exercises, diet, and meditation. When the moment of birth comes, she is not drugged and immobilized on an operating table, as is customary in the West. After birth she is not left half-drugged with an empty feeling, and prevented from touching and holding her own new child.

Learning Without Strain

Just like kittens, little children are naturally curious. They want to know about important things. They keep pestering their parents with "silly questions." They want to know where we come from, why the sky is blue, why grown-ups smoke cigarettes, why some things float in the bathtub while others sink, why girls are different from boys, why rainbows are colorful, and why they have to go to bed at night. This is what biology, physics, chemistry, history,

---

[6] Frederick Leboyer, *Birth without Violence* (New York: Alfred Knopf, 1975).

and other school subjects are all about. Nothing could make children happier than to have these things explained to them, at their own level and at their own rate of progress.

Children also learn by following the example of those whom they love and admire. They automatically reject the knowledge that comes from people whom they dislike. What they learn from most teachers at school under duress is grudgingly memorized, but it does not really become integrated into their store of practical and useful knowledge. After a few years of coercive schooling they have lost their natural urge to acquire essential facts and to use their minds creatively.

That learning can be fun and that teaching can be done without coercion has been proven by the many schools established by A. S. Neill, Rudolf Steiner, and others. As soon as teachers learn to present the material in interesting ways, most pupils consider going to school a privilege and a pleasure.

It has been found that children who attend such free schools become more creative, self-motivated, self-reliant, and responsible in later life. They learn more easily and know how to gather relevant information. They are more kind and other-oriented, and ready to help with community activities.

Not everything in life can be fun, of course, and children should also be shown the value of patience, hard work, and discipline. They must know how to strive and compete when necessary, and to endure temporary mental and physical strain. But to make them strain habitually day after day and year after year only frustrates them and turns them into unbalanced or neurotic adults. They can no longer think and act spontaneously from the center. They do not know that the human mind and body are most efficient and successful when they function naturally and joyfully.

CHAPTER 17

Everything Falls into Place

The All-Encompassing Dan-Tien Experience

When we are not centered in the Dan-Tien, everything becomes an effort, and nothing works quite right. We notice this not only in practical everyday life, but in all other areas of our world, in our social life, love life, work, health, religion, politics, etc. But when we find the balance again, everything suddenly makes sense, and the pieces of the puzzle fall into place.

We can now paint a picture of how we think and feel when we live in touch with the Dan-Tien, with regard to mind and body, intellect and intuition, conscious and unconscious mind, theory and practice, activity and rest, thoughts and feelings, male and female, father and mother, right and left, culture and nature, etc.

Signs of a Centered Life

We benefit from a continuous creative interplay between thoughts and feelings. Our subconscious mind becomes a friend and a source of vital energy and inspiration. We are on good terms

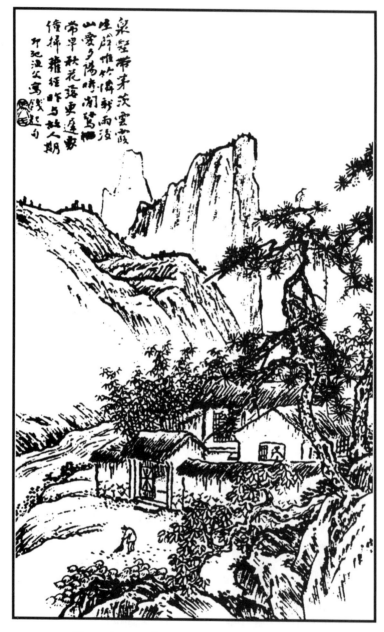

Figure 25. We function in tune with nature and we have access to the cosmic life energy.

with the body and feel at home in it. We know that mental and physical health go hand in hand. We are seldom troubled by psychosomatic ills, and we experience the bodily functions as pleasant. Therefore we seek out healers who cooperate with the body and know how to mobilize its inherent healing forces, instead of coercing it with chemicals and surgery.

We are in touch with our inner as well as our outer world, and we know how to harmonize the two. We function in tune with nature instead of against it and we have access to the cosmic life energy. We can quickly recover from periods of strain or illness.

We know that theory and practice are two sides of a coin, that they complement and enhance each other. We adjust the theory whenever it turns out to be impractical, and we improve our practice by paying attention to theory. We get practical results without forgetting our principles.

We know how to create "Heaven on Earth" in this life, by harmonizing heavenly and earthly qualities within us and around us, right here and now. Although we have high ideals, we have both feet on the ground. We have sublime aspirations, and we also enjoy the blessings of Mother Earth.

Although we appreciate the benefits of culture, we are only interested in the type of culture that harmonizes with nature. We prefer a way of life that is cultured in a natural way. We feel good in natural surroundings, surrounded by plants and animals. Being products of nature ourselves, we like to see culture as a highly evolved expression of nature.

We know that men and women are made to appreciate each other, that they complement each other in their respective functions. They are two sides of a coin, and they each have their strong and weak points. Both of them are "good" when they harmonize with each other, and both of them show their negative or vicious sides when this harmony is lost. We see the same polarity in the relation between father and mother, each having their respective vital functions in bringing up children.

We realize that the mind functions best when right and left brain hemispheres harmonize. With respect to right and left in politics we know that both sides of the political spectrum have their valid functions, that both of them are needed in a healthy community. We need to cultivate both private and communal goals and interests. In the ideal society, individual and social enterprise coincide for mutual benefit. Neither pure socialism nor pure private capitalism can offer all the answers and satisfy all human needs.

When it comes to the relation between government and people, we know that they each have their vital functions, their strong and weak points. The government is responsible for coordinating and defending the community, and the people set the general tone and provide material support.

In the same way we realize that we need our Dan-Tien to set the general tone in everything we think and do, and that we need our head to deal with the details and the world around us.

We know from experience that we attain all these benefits automatically when we feel good in the Dan-Tien. To know this we do not need faith in a theory or belief. At any given moment we can prove to ourselves that the Dan-Tien is there and that it works wonders if we let it.

The Meaning of Life

Human beings need to feel that their life has meaning. Without meaning life soon becomes sad or even unbearable. If they experience their own and other people's lives as meaningless they cannot be happy as individuals or as members of society.

When we live in tune with the cosmic life energy through the Dan-Tien, everything we think and do gains meaning. Everything around us and within us seems to be pervaded by Chi, and life seems to have a cosmic purpose. This is not a belief or faith, but a spontaneous experience.

But as soon as we lose touch with the Dan-Tien, we feel lost in a meaningless universe. "The mass of men lead lives of quiet desperation," said Henry David Thoreau.[1] Victor Frankl describes

---

[1] Henry David Thoreau, *The Portable Thoreau* (London: Penguin, 1977), "Economy," p. 263.

in his *Man's Search for Meaning* that a person's survival in desperate conditions depends on his/her belief in the meaning of life.[2]

Because such a belief is so vital, people often cling desperately to any faith or theory, however irrational, as long as it seems to give their life some meaning. The history books and newspapers are full of examples.

Poor people may think that getting rich is the purpose of life. When, after years of struggling, they have a home, two cars, and three bank accounts, they feel no happier and turn to alcohol or drugs. Young people may feel that growing up is the purpose of life. But when they grow up, they find life just as meaningless. Not long ago the desperate masses in many countries clung to ideologies that promised a glorious destiny through fascism or communism. Throughout history people have blindly believed those who claimed to know the word of God and the meaning of life, especially if this served their own selfish interests. Hindus in India believe that life is a painful illusion, and they yearn to be liberated from this life and future incarnations. Many parents suffer and struggle through life, merely to have children who suffer and struggle to have children, and so on.

But when people discover the secret of Dan-Tien, they experience meaning in everything they think and do. Each minute finds fulfillment in itself. Each minute is a little treasure that connects them with the source of life and is theirs forever.

---

[2] Victor Frankl, *Man's Search for Meaning* (New York: Simon & Schuster, 1984).

Bibliography

Benedict, Ruth. *Patterns of Culture.* New York. 1935.

Bolen, Jean Shinoda. *The Tao of Psychology.* New York: Harper & Row, 1979.

Brown, Barbara B.: *New Mind, New Body.* New York: Harper & Row, 1974.

Calthorpe, Peter. "Pedestrian Pockets." *Whole Earth Review,* Spring 1988.

Campbell, Joseph. *Myths to Live By.* New York: Bantam Books, 1988.

Chia, Mantak. *Taoist Ways to Transform Stress into Vitality.* Huntington, NY: Healing Tao, 1986.

Diamond, John. *Your Body Doesn't Lie.* New York: Warner, 1989.

Dürkheim, Karlfried Graf. *Hara.* New York: Fernhill House, 1970.

Dychtwald, Ken. *Body-Mind.* New York: Jove/Pantheon, 1977.

Emerson, Ralph Waldo. *Emerson's Essays.* New York: HarperCollins, 1981.

Frankl, Victor. *Man's Search for Meaning.* New York: Touchstone, 1984.

Gallwey, W. Timothy. *The Inner Game of Golf.* New York: Random, 1981.

———. *The Inner Game of Tennis.* New York: Bantam, 1984.

Gawain, Shakti. *Creative Visualization*. New York: Bantam Books, 1983.

Hay, Louise. *You Can Heal Your Life*. Los Angeles: Hay House, 1987.

Heider, John. *The Tao of Leadership*. New York: Bantam Books, 1986.

Herrigel, Eugen. *Zen in the Art of Archery*. New York: Vintage Books, 1971.

Hoff, Benjamin. *The Tao of Pooh*. New York: Viking/Penguin, 1983.

I Ching or Book of Changes, Richard Wilhelm translation, rendered into English by Gary F. Baynes. Foreword by C. G. Jung, Bollingen Series XIX. New York: Pantheon Books for the Bollingen Foundation, 1950.

Keleman, Stanley. *Your Body Speaks Its Mind*. New York: Simon & Schuster, 1976.

Kurtz, Ron. *The Body Reveals*. New York: Harper & Row, 1976.

Lao Tzu. *Tao Te Ching*. D. C. Lau, trans. London: Penguin, 1963.

Leboyer, Frederick. *Birth without Violence*. New York: A. Knopf, 1975.

Liedloff, Jean. *The Continuum Concept*. Reading, MA: Addison Wesley, 1985.

Long, Barry. *Ridding Yourself of Unhappiness*. London: Barry Long Foundation, 1987.

Lowen, Alexander. *Betrayal of the Body*. New York: Collier Books, 1967.

———. *Bioenergetics*. New York: Viking/Penguin, 1976.

Markert, Christopher. *I Ching: The Ultimate Success Formula*. London: Aquarian Press, 1986.

———. *Seeing Well Again*. Saffron Walden, England: C.W. Daniel, 1982 and Englewood Cliffs, NJ: Prentice Hall, 1983.

Maslow, Abraham. *Toward a Psychology of Being*. New York: Van Nos Reinhold, 1968.

Masters, Robert. *Listening to the Body*. New York: Delta Publishing, 1978.

Mendelsohn, Robert, MD. *Confessions of a Medical Heretic.* Chicago: Contemporary Books, 1979.

Nara, Robert O. *Dental Self-Sufficiency.* Lake Linder, MI: Oramedics, 1975 (R.R.1, Box 112, zip 49945).

Selye, Hans. *The Stress of Life.* New York: McGraw-Hill, 1956.

Yutang, Lin. *The Importance of Living.* London: Wm. Heinemann Ltd., 1938.

Index

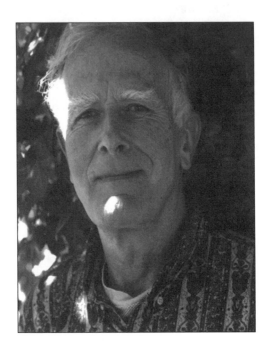

Christopher J. Markert (70) immigrated to the USA from Germany, where he had studied sociology at Munich University and worked in public opinion research at the Institut für Demoskopie. In New York he joined Young and Rubicam (an advertising agency), then Raymond Loewy Associates (industrial design), and later a division of the McGraw-Hill Publishing Company in San Francisco. In 1970 his first book was published, *Test Your Emotions,* which sold over 700,000 copies in nine countries, including the USA. In recent years he has written four books about the practical aspects of Far-Eastern wisdom. In his present work, *Dan-Tien—Your Secret Energy Center,* he shows how we can make the best of each day by living in tune with our inner source of vitality and joy.